MEET
your
KARMA

About the Author

For two decades Shelley A. Kaehr, PhD, has worked with thousands of people around the world, helping them achieve greater peace and happiness in their lives.

Her past life regression process has been endorsed by Dr. Brian Weiss, who called her work "an important contribution to the field of regression therapy."

A world traveler, Shelley believes the soul longs to return to places from prior incarnations. She coined the term *Supretrovie* to describe sudden recollections of prior lives while traveling, and she believes all people, whether they consciously remember it or not, have flashbacks from prior lives while going about their daily business.

Shelley received her PhD in Parapsychic Science from the American Institute of Holistic Theology in 2001. She is a Certified Clinical Hypnotherapist and Trainer and lives near Dallas, Texas. She truly believes we all have the ability to make positive changes and live the life of our dreams.

Visit Shelley online:

https://pastlifelady.com

Facebook Fan Page: Past Life Lady

Instagram: shelleykaehr

YouTube: Past Life Lady

Twitter: @ShelleyKaehr

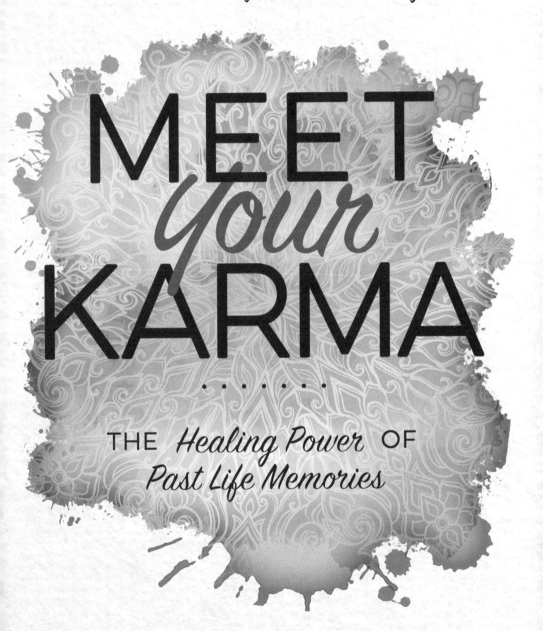

CLEAR YOUR
Anxiety, Depression, & Trauma
THROUGH *Self-Guided Journeys*

MEET *your* KARMA

·······

THE *Healing Power* OF
Past Life Memories

SHELLEY A. KAEHR, PhD

LLEWELLYN PUBLICATIONS
WOODBURY, MINNESOTA

First Edition
First Printing, 2020

Book design by Samantha Penn
Cover design by Shannon McKuhen

Llewellyn Publications is a registered trademark of Llewellyn Worldwide Ltd.

Library of Congress Cataloging-in-Publication Data
Names: Kaehr, Shelley, author.
Title: Meet your karma : the healing power of past life memories / Shelley
    A. Kaehr, PhD.
Description: First edition. | Woodbury, Minnesota : Llewellyn
    Publications, 2020. | Includes bibliographical references.
Identifiers: LCCN 2019043438 (print) | LCCN 2019043439 (ebook) | ISBN
    9780738762173 (paperback) | ISBN 9780738762234 (ebook)
Subjects: LCSH: Reincarnation. | Reincarnation—Case studies.
Classification: LCC BL515 .K335 2020 (print) | LCC BL515 (ebook) | DDC
    133.901/35—dc23
LC record available at https://lccn.loc.gov/2019043438
LC ebook record available at https://lccn.loc.gov/2019043439

Llewellyn Worldwide Ltd. does not participate in, endorse, or have any authority or responsibility concerning private business transactions between our authors and the public.

All mail addressed to the author is forwarded but the publisher cannot, unless specifically instructed by the author, give out an address or phone number.

Any internet references contained in this work are current at publication time, but the publisher cannot guarantee that a specific location will continue to be maintained. Please refer to the publisher's website for links to authors' websites and other sources.

Llewellyn Publications
A Division of Llewellyn Worldwide Ltd.
2143 Wooddale Drive
Woodbury, MN 55125-2989
www.llewellyn.com

Printed in the United States of America

Other Books by Shelley A. Kaehr, PhD

Past Lives with Pets

Lifestream: Journey into Past & Future Lives

Supretrovie: Externally Induced Past Life Memories

Familiar Places: Reflections on Past Lives Around the World

Reincarnation Recollections: Geographically Induced Past Life Memories

Past Lives with Gems & Stones

This book is dedicated to the thousands of people I've had the privilege to work with through the years and to all truth-seekers. May you find true happiness, peace, and joy in your current life and forevermore.

Contents

Exercises

Disclaimer

This book is not intended as a substitute for consultation with a licensed medical or mental health professional. The reader should regularly consult a physician or mental health professional in matters relating to his/her health and particularly with respect to any symptoms that may require diagnosis or medical attention. This book provides content related to educational, medical, and psychological topics. As such, use of this book implies your acceptance of this disclaimer.

Some names and identifying details have been changed to protect the privacy of individuals.

Acknowledgments

This book is dedicated to the thousands of souls I've had the privilege of working with throughout my career, and to all who seek to discover deep meaning from their past. With any project of this magnitude, I could not have completed this book without the help of a huge team of people, and the loving support from friends and family. I owe an enormous debt of gratitude to Angela Wix, who believed in the project from the beginning and without whom this book would not exist. To Bill Krause, Terry Lohmann, Kat Sanborn, Jake-Ryan Kent, Annie Burdick, Lynne Menturweck, Patti Frazee, Sami Sherratt, Leah Madsen, Sammy Penn, Shannon McKuhen, Anna Levine and the rest of the incredible team at Llewellyn, I am eternally grateful for your support. Special thanks and kudos to my family and friends, including Jim Merideth, Pat Moon, Paula Wagner, and Karen Wiley.

Introduction

I MET MY KARMA the moment I came into this world kicking and scream-ing. I was healthy at birth, but at two and a half weeks old I suddenly became gravely ill. Doctors said my kidneys had shut down for no apparent reason and told my parents to brace for the worst. A month into my hospital stay, the doctors sent me home to die. On a soul level, I didn't seem particularly thrilled to be here this time. Then my grandmother suddenly passed away and a miracle happened: All my vitals inexplicably returned to normal. The kidney diagnosis could never be proven. Once I recovered, doctors found no clinical evidence that anything was ever wrong with me at all.

Years later when I became a professional past life regression therapist, I discovered that in my most recent incarnation before this one I was an alco-holic drug addict, born in the 1940s, and died in the 1960s of kidney failure. I came screeching right back into mortality in 1967 because I had some tough lessons to learn and things to do here in this lifetime.

Astrologically speaking, I was born with the Sun in my sixth house, which is not ideal for health. While astrology offers a good roadmap of what we come here as souls to work on, I managed to overcome all of these challenges with a combination of past life regression, energy work, and meditation—all of the methods you will read about in this book.

My belief in reincarnation started in childhood, after my mother attended a luncheon with guest speaker Virginia Tighe, the subject of one of the most famous past life regression cases in history, *The Search for Bridey Murphy*. If you're not familiar with this book, Tighe suffered from severe allergies and explored several remedies but nothing worked, so she tried hypnosis. Regressing back to her childhood helped some but never completely resolved the problem. The frustrated hypnotherapist finally asked her to go back to the *source event* where her allergies first started. To everyone's surprise, she zipped back into her former incarnation in nineteenth-century Ireland, where she recounted incredibly specific details about her life as Bridey Murphy.

That night after the luncheon at our family dinner table, my parents and I discussed the validity of past lives. From that moment on, I believed in reincarnation. The idea made complete sense to me. I had never accepted that we only live a short hundred years or less on Earth and then simply vanish into the cosmic dust of heaven, where our souls linger for all eternity.

As an adult, my belief in reincarnation strengthened after a friend died in a hiking accident during a trip on which I'd been invited but declined to go. The situation caused years of regret and constant rehashing of dozens of unproductive *what if*-type scenarios. After years of traditional therapy, trying to heal and release my unresolved grief, I had no luck whatsoever. Eventually, someone suggested I try past life regression. The regression instantly changed my life for the better. I learned my friend and I had shared many past lives together in which he had died too young.

Our souls have contracts to fulfill, all things happen for a reason, and witnessing these truths under hypnosis gave me a deeper personal experience of the fact that we are indeed moving on from here to a better place after death.

The regression solidified my commitment to spend my life bringing this kind of relief to others through the power of past life journeys. Finding the root cause alleviates needless suffering. More importantly, you can often come to a place of acceptance of some of life's tougher lessons.

I found this out in 2000, when I attended my first hypnotherapy training class. During the course, we spent a month giving and receiving sessions in order to become certified. This was excruciatingly painful, to say the least. I had a lot of heavy karma energetically bogging me down.

I had just returned to Texas after a painful divorce, and during that agony, I had willed myself to leave my body. I journeyed into the tunnel of light Raymond Moody talks about in his book *Life After Life*. Basically, I was finished. I did not want to live anymore. Not simply because of the divorce, but more from a heavy, overwhelming feeling of failure.

When I showed up in Texas, I was broken. Not really, of course, but I felt that way. When I went into the light, I met with some of my dead relatives, including the grandmother who had died right after I was born and whom I'd never known in life. I will never forget what a surprise it was to see her standing there. She told me it was not my time. I returned from the light and went back into my body. I felt hypersensitive to light, sound, and energy. I could not work. I had to take a break from life for a while, but as I am not one to sit around twiddling my thumbs, I decided to take the hypnotherapy class instead.

I had no idea how much stuff would be dredged up from not only my past lives but my current life past. It was unbelievably emotional. I emerged from the training feeling ten thousand times better than I'd ever felt before in my current life. I realized without a doubt that you actually have to go *through* negative emotions to overcome them. Avoiding them altogether only causes the body to break down and become weak. Releasing negative emotions strengthens the soul, because once that stuck energy is gone, new light becomes available to you and your whole life can change in a flash.

Hypnotic journeys freed me in a major way and showed me that there is nothing to be afraid of in confronting the past. Hypnosis and past life regression allow you to see events from a new perspective; they lighten your spirit and free you to enjoy your current life more fully. Once I figured this out, I made it my mission to help other people break through the bonds of material existence to find greater joy in life.

Through my own experiences, and after spending the past twenty years in private practice working with over three thousand clients, I know for a fact that many of our current life difficulties are direct carryovers from situations that originated well beyond and before our current lifetime. As such, with proper guidance, anyone can overcome even the toughest diagnosis. I've done it myself, and I've seen miracles happen to lots of other people.

I've had an incredibly diverse clientele over the years, specializing in a unique blend of hypnosis and energy healing. I found that our thoughts really do occupy physical space in the unseen energy fields around our bodies, and likewise, our past life memories also exist in unseen yet physical form. My methods address issues on both the verbal cognitive level and energetically so my clients can achieve lasting change. I discovered that it's not enough to clear things out by talking them through. Memories must be cleared energetically so the issue remains resolved. Using the power of their imaginations, I guide my clients to revisit past incarnations, receive their lessons, and use that knowledge to empower their current lives.

The other major aspect of my work involves what I call *future memories.* Clients visit their current-life futures so they can see themselves successful and happy, living the life they truly want. Quantum physics has proven time is illusory at best, so the higher purpose for revising our past is to empower our current life. Clients experience their highest potential firsthand, because that probability exists in the realm of the quantum field as surely as any other. I wrote *Meet Your Karma* because of my concerns about the staggering increase in anxiety, trauma, and depression rampant in today's society. Thanks to technology, we are becoming increasingly isolated from our fellow beings, and, sadly, we are only now beginning to see the long-term consequences of being stuck on our devices. According to the Centers for Disease Control (CDC), suicide is now the tenth leading cause of death in America,[1] a statistic that disturbs me deeply. Although there are now a wide variety of medicinal treatments to help alleviate suffering, unfortunately they aren't helping everyone.

That's one of the main reasons why people come to see me. I'm quite often the last resort, the final straw when all else fails and people are left asking themselves what they're missing in terms of finding the root cause of certain chronic situations. People suffering from depression, anxiety, and trauma often bring those conditions straight over from past lives, and in some cases, I can help. My intent for this book is to help you uncover and heal your own traumas and anxieties, give you tools and strategies for coping with daily life, and through a series of case histories, hopefully make you realize you are far from alone in your struggles.

How to Use This Book

This book is divided into three sections. Part one will discuss the philosophical aspects of reincarnation. Part two will reveal fascinating case histories of clients who demonstrated various symptoms of stress, anxiety, depression,

. . . .

1. NCHS, National Vital Statistics System, Mortality. Figure 4: "Age-adjusted death rates for the 10 leading causes of death: United States, 2016 and 2017," CDC.gov. https://www.cdc.gov/nchs/products/databriefs/db328.htm.

trauma, and other disorders identified by the American Psychiatric Associ-ations Diagnostic Statistics Manual (DSM). While most of the clients you'll read about have not necessarily been clinically diagnosed with these disor-ders, the case histories I'm including show the breadth of conditions and challenges that can be successfully remedied with past life regression therapy. Finally, in part three, I will share my RELIEF Method for anxiety, depres-sion, and trauma. I developed this acronym (RELIEF) to describe the vari-ous stages my clients go through during the hypnotic process. You will have the opportunity to experience the RELIEF method for yourself through a series of progressive, guided journeys that I pray will provide you with insight, answers, and healing.

PART ONE
· · · · ·
Past Lives, Regression, & the RELIEF Method

A 2018 PEW RESEARCH Center survey found 33 percent of American adults now believe in reincarnation.[2] That seems like a small number when you consider the millions of other people around the globe who accept past lives as truth. Still, the number of people in the United States who are more open to this idea has certainly increased since I started working in this field twenty years ago.

Before delving into case histories, I will discuss some of the philosophical aspects of past life regression and why it's not necessary to believe in reincarnation in order for regressions to work. I'll also share common reasons for seeking regression and some of the amazing benefits you can experience from using this modality.

· · · · · · · · · · · ·
2. Claire Gecewicz, "'New Age' Beliefs Common Among Religious, Nonreligious Americans." Pew Research Center, October 1, 2018. http://www.pewresearch.org/fact-tank/2018/10/01/new-age-beliefs-common-among-both-religious-and-nonreligious-americans/.

CHAPTER 1
. . . .

Past Lives &
Regression

THERE HAVE ALWAYS BEEN doubters who do not believe in past lives. That's fine. All belief systems have critics. Renowned philosopher Carl Jung thought humankind shares a collective unconscious where all the memories of the human species are stored. Certain symbolic figures, or archetypes, are universal in nature, and all people, regardless of background, understand them. Heroes and villains, mothers and wise old men, are among the examples of archetypal energies that are universal in our society. Some believe when people go on hypnotic journeys, it is quite possible they are simply tapping into the archetypal shared past of the ancestors, rather than venturing back in time to their own personal memories.

When I guide my clients into the past and ask certain questions, incredibly, they always give an answer. Where do those answers come from? There's no way to know for sure, although I believe the data bubbles up from the depths of the soul. I can't say with absolute certainty that these memories are real. I do not claim to understand the inner workings of the Universe. Some people may have lived before, while others may simply be escaping into a world they saw on TV, while others may have succeeded in tapping into the universal mind.

Whatever the case, in my mind, the hypnotic journey worked if positive results are achieved. Any time I assist clients with anxiety, stress, depression, or trauma, the main goal is to help them find relief. I am not busy googling or fact-checking everything they say, because that is not the most important aspect of the work. What matters, *all that matters*, is helping someone increase overall happiness and tranquility in their life.

Belief Systems

On that note, this is a great time to bring up belief systems. If you're reading this book, then you either believe in reincarnation or you're exploring the idea. While reincarnation is a religious belief for Hindus, Buddhists, and others, in the context of what we're talking about in *Meet Your Karma*, past life regression is not a belief, it's a *process*. I believe we have lived before and we will be back again, and yet I am not endorsing a religion here, nor am I insisting you change your personal belief systems. In fact, you don't actually have to believe in past lives to benefit from past life regression. You'll see examples of this in part two when you read the case studies.

You may be like so many of my clients who find themselves struggling with the model of the world they grew up in and the things their parents and other authority figures taught them, and how to integrate new thoughts and feelings that contradict what they've been raised to believe is right or wrong. That feeling is perfectly normal and understandable. The idea of reincarnation is a construct of humankind, and therefore there is no way to prove or disprove past lives.

In Western culture, many Christians were raised to believe that reincarnation either does not exist at all, or it's evil to consider, even though evidence suggests that at one time, the Bible mentioned reincarnation before it was removed.

Interestingly, a 2018 Pew Research Center survey showed that while Christians may not admit their true beliefs publicly, 29 percent of Christians actually do believe in reincarnation.[3] Most of my clients identify as Christian. Perhaps this is due to the thinning of the veils, so to speak; the new onslaught of readily available materials and knowledge that was once not-so-accessible

· · · · · · · · · · · ·

3. Gecewicz, "'New Age' Beliefs Common Among Religious, Nonreligious Americans."

has us asking more questions about our origins and the meaning of life more than ever. The mixing of theoretically opposite beliefs could also be a result of people not finding satisfactory answers to deeper questions about our purpose for being.

Why Do a Past Life Regression?

Bringing balance to life in mind, body, and spirit is a lifelong challenge. When any of these areas is out of alignment, people search for answers to help restore stability in their lives. Past life regression is an amazing self-discovery tool for anything you can think of, including the following.

1. Love & Relationships

We all want someone to love and we want to feel like we're a part of something beyond ourselves, be it family, friends, church, or spiritual community. We want to belong. When we're having difficulty in our relationship and have tried regular means to alleviate the issue, sometimes a past life is at the core. The subconscious patterns and behaviors we act out with various people can be uncovered by going into past life situations and taking note of how the relationships we have in our current life are the same or different from how they used to be hundreds of years ago. Many times, you can easily notice that you've been doing the same things with the same people again and again, and that realization can create an incredible epiphany and lead to healing and transformation so a relationship can become more of what you want. If needed, a regression can give you the strength to release situations that are no longer serving you because they haven't been working for longer than you consciously realized.

I cannot begin to tell you how many sessions I've done for people struggling with challenges involving the people in their lives. Face it, relationships are often tough and bring both the most lessons and the most learning about ourselves. One of the big causes for anxiety and stress has always been relationships, and regressions are incredibly informative to help you gain new insights into yourself and others. Regression can uncover hidden information about:

Romantic Love: Challenges with romance are some of the main reasons people have a regression. How did you know your loved one in the past? The exploration could be good or bad—either this connection is so awesome, you know you've known him or her for years, or things have gone south fast and now you want answers. Either way, regression works!

Family Love: Regardless of your background, family is a major source of karma. Analyzing underlying dynamics that either bind your family together or tear you apart can be incredibly helpful information. Regression also provides clues on how to improve your current-life relationships by looking for answers in your past.

Friendship Love: I believe we travel with our friends through many lifetimes and the people closest to us, those who have our backs, have often been in that role before. Haven't you met someone and become fast friends for reasons that defy explanation? And when you're apart, sometimes for years on end, when you reunite, it's like time stands still and you pick up where you left off? That's a friend for *lives*!

Self-Love: While relationships with others provide an experience of love, you can also learn about self-love through acceptance and forgiveness by seeing that all trials we go through are gifts to help us grow. Oftentimes we are far easier on people around us than we are on ourselves. Past life regression helps us look at our lives from a new vantage point so we can easily identify the reasons behind challenges and the lessons learned.

I am a big believer that we came into our current lifetime having already planned out our lessons before we arrived. What we do for soul growth can often be deepened by going into past life experiences where perhaps our soul learned the same or similar lessons.

Other Challenging Relationships: Whether you're having difficulties with a boss or being bullied at school, these challenges can be addressed, and often better understood, after undergoing regression. When you don't get along with someone for any apparent reason, or you have a bad vibe about a person without them even opening their mouth, the past can often be the source. When you find the originating point of the challenge and work to bring healing to the relationship, you can transform a challenge into a true blessing.

2. Health

You don't always notice your health until it's deteriorated. If you are too ill to get out of bed, then all other areas of life suddenly don't matter anymore. Both physical and emotional health is critical to our well-being. Health is another cause of anxiety and stress. When we're facing a physical crisis, emotional stress follows. Particularly with chronic conditions, often there is an emotional core, a source event that can be identified in past lives that can bring healing to the current situation. Regression can never replace common sense or medical treatment, but it can relieve the trauma and anxiety that are often residual side effects of life-threatening situations.

You can also visit the energetic source of a health challenge in order to heal and transform the illness or *dis-ease* at the root. Oftentimes when nothing else works to fully alleviate a health crisis, a regression can assist you with neutralizing the emotional undercurrent of the illness.

When my friend died years ago, my depression caused my health to deteriorate, and I received true relief from past life regression, as have countless others.

3. Money

Call it what you want—money, security, having a roof over your head—if you lack security in the material world and are having a hard time looking past your next paycheck—or, for some, the next meal—stress, anxiety, and depression will follow. Believe it or not, the relationship we have with money is deeply embedded in our souls and is heavily influenced by our early experiences in our current life, by how we were raised and what our parents believed. People often attempt to resolve money issues by working on healing the triggers or changing the beliefs instilled in them by well-meaning caregivers; however, sometimes this won't work if the key to the difficulty originated in past lives.

Many times, the relationship with money is like dealing with a person. We've been doing the same things over and over again, expecting a different result, but we are not consciously aware of those prior lifetimes where things were tough. By traveling into the past and doing some transformative work, you can make great headway on this issue that plagues so many people today and find new solutions to alter your thinking and increase your bottom line by shifting to a mindset of abundance and prosperity.

4. Making an Impact & Higher Purpose

If you're reading this book, I would bet you have a deep desire to make your life mean something and to have a tangible impact on your fellow beings. Often the desire for higher purpose is clearer than the way to achieve that goal. Past life regression reveals our soul's mission in a way few other modalities can, because you can peek into your deep past, find your hidden or underutilized gifts and talents, and enliven them toward your utmost potential. I've seen people suffering from intense anxiety because on some deeper level they believed they had a higher purpose that they were not quite reaching. The memory is stuck so deep in the subconscious goo, they can't let it out. Regression helps you do just that, so you can live up to your full potential and find greater happiness in life.

5. Adventure

Many people are highly motivated by a sense of adventure and the zest to go out into our wonderful world and experience all life has to offer. I coined a term, *Supretrovie* (based on French terms for supernatural past life), which are spontaneous past life memories triggered by travel, artifacts, or other external stimuli. I've talked to hundreds of people who did not need hypnosis but were reminded about their past lives simply by traveling to a new place. I am absolutely convinced that we are spiritually called to visit locations where we've lived in prior incarnations. Our soul longs to re-experience the comfort and familiarity of the places we've loved in the past, and our souls want to heal trauma from times long gone when things did not go as well as we'd hoped. Those who seek adventure and want to see the world often discover that a regression deepens their appreciation for the world we live in and the reasons why we are drawn to the people, places, and things that we love.

6. Curiosity

This is surprisingly one of the most common reasons people want a session. They've been hearing about past life regression on the news more often these days, or they saw a documentary on the *Lifetime* network and now they want to know if they've had past lives. You will see in the case study section of this book that curiosity leads some to see me for a regression, but it's interesting to note that oftentimes people uncover the source of trauma and anxiety during the session. The truth is, there are no coincidences or accidents in our universe. At some level, the client's subconscious mind, along with my intent for them to go to events that are for their highest good, often guides people to uncover incredibly transformational material that completely shifts their lives around for the better, simply because they were curious about the process. At a higher level, their soul had a plan far greater than the conscious mind realized.

7. Healing/Forgiving

Healing and forgiving encompasses a wide variety of situations, ranging from releasing anger and resentment toward a family member to trying to move past feelings of grief, loss, and loneliness after the death of a lost loved one or locating the source event of an illness, and everything in between. All healing involves willingness to let go of the negativity of the past and move into a brighter tomorrow. No doubt, if we harbor resentments and angst about troubling times in our current past, we're on the road to deep anxiety. Past life regression powerfully resolves such situations, as you will soon discover.

8. Remembering

One of my favorite reasons to take people on a regression journey is to help people remember who they are as souls. We all have natural abilities that come easily to us, and visiting our past sheds valuable light on where latent talents lie so you capitalize on your gifts in your current lifetime.

I've found that almost anything you can think of that you'd like to know about yourself can be addressed by undergoing a past life regression. The wellspring of information can be truly transformational, and because there are no accidents in the universe, the information needed will be revealed to you at a beneficial time on your life's journey.

How Past Life Regression Works

Here are a few thoughts about why past life regression works so well.

Associated versus Dissociated

When you go through events in real life, you view them through your own eyes and are completely *associated* in the event. When you go back in time via hypnosis, you view such events either from a new perspective, such as floating over events and looking down on them as if watching actors on a stage, or it can look like viewing the scene on a movie or laptop screen. This distanced vision is considered *dissociated*, and from that perspective, you can gain new perspective and relief.

Rewinding a Film

According to modern psychology, your short-term memory can only hold up to seven chunks of data at any given time.[4] Think about that for a moment, and you'll realize it's true. If I ask you a specific question, you can go into your memory bank, find the answer and bring it up to the forefront of your mind so you can tell me the answer, but there is definitely a searching process that goes on before the memory is retrieved.

Every single thing you have ever witnessed in any lifetime is stored within the depths of your subconscious mind, which is like a priceless storehouse of video recordings of every single thing your soul has ever done in all of your lifetimes. The challenge is to rewind these internal videos of memories and return to the originating incident where the issue first began. Theoretically, the source event could have happened yesterday, when you were a child, or anything in between. When searching those current life memories doesn't yield the results you want, that's when it's time to go further back, well beyond conscious awareness to your past lives.

. . . .

4. G. Miller, "The magical number seven, plus or minus two: Some limits on our capacity for processing information." *The Psychological Review* 63: 81–97, 1956.

Why We Don't Remember

You do not consciously recall your past life experiences because, typically, most souls agree to dip into what the ancient Greeks called the River of Forgetfulness. When you incarnated in a body, you decided on a soul level to participate in the school of life by learning various prearranged lessons that would help you mature as a soul. Part of why this growth is so profound is the fact that you agreed to forget all that happened to you in prior lifetimes so you could enjoy a challenging path of self-discovery.

Conscious vs. Subconscious Mind

You have two aspects to your consciousness—your conscious mind and sub-conscious mind. The conscious mind handles day-to-day life, and is comprised of your ego, or how to identify yourself and the world around you in the three-dimensional space.

Your subconscious mind is the storehouse for these memories we've been discussing. Unlike the collective unconscious mentioned earlier, the sub-conscious handles storing your personal memories and information, rather than that of the entire society. The other reason you forget your past lives is because your subconscious mind believes that recalling trauma would be detrimental to you in the long run, so in order to keep you "safe" it represses unpleasant memories, hiding them away deep in the inexhaustible storehouse of your mind. To a certain extent, that's a good thing. If we were continually bombarded by negativity all the time, it would be incredibly difficult to get through a day, let alone a lifetime.

The challenge comes when too much repressed memory begins to over-flow and bubble up into waking reality, manifesting into anything from physical illness to anxiety or depression.

When unexpressed emotions linger under the surface of our psyches, eventually illness and *dis-ease* can result. The body will find a way to expel these energies and often the results are incredibly unpleasant. Believe me, I know. I've been there.

When my friend died many years ago, I decided to ignore the grief until my health began to decline and I could not do so any longer. My journey is the reason why I became a healer and hypnotherapist in the first place. Once

I delved into my suppressed emotions and realized that they were nothing to fear, I finally began to heal physically, emotionally, and spiritually.

The strange paradox of fear is that we believe it will be horrible to relive something and that if we do, it won't go away. Actually, the exact opposite is true. Once you bring up something unpleasant, you can reframe and heal the negativity, and then the old memory actually goes away. Stuffing things down, however, ensures that whatever we don't acknowledge will haunt us.

A good example of this is my client Carol, who had an unexplained fear and panicked whenever she approached a tunnel either in a car or on a train. During her first regression, she claimed she didn't see anything, but later she admitted, "I had a flash of being in a tunnel, and then everything went black."

Many people claim they don't see anything when they take a hypnotic journey, even though they often later admit that tiny flashes of insight came through. They either dismiss those epiphanies as nonsense, or refuse to expound on the details in the session. Why does this happen? Because the subconscious mind suppresses information until you're ready to receive it. Hidden memories emerge on a need-to-know basis.

I know this firsthand because this happened to me during my first past life regression. I saw a brief flash of a pair of cowboy boots on a dusty road, and nothing more. Several years later, when I had my second regression, that initial scene opened up and I had a total experience about that lifetime where I received incredibly helpful information, which I will share with you later in the book. Why does this happen? Along with our subconscious minds, our spirit guides and our own Higher Self will not allow us to open doorways we're not meant to open. Plus, our human consciousness is like an onion, so as we peel back more and more layers of this onion of consciousness, we will get answers and insights when we are ready and not a moment before, which is why there is nothing to fear from having a regression.

Another reason why you're always safe in hypnosis is because during the hypnotic journey, your brainwaves slow down from the waking state, called beta, down into the alpha or theta states, which access healing and suppressed memories. During all of these processes, you are in total control of your emotions, you have an ability to stop at any time, and you are able to access lost chunks of data easier than when you're fully awake, because slowing your brainwaves down actually brings you a heightened sense of awareness.

Later in the book I will tell you what happened when Carol fully explored her fear of tunnels at a time when her Higher Self finally felt ready to receive that information. For now, just know that I've seen a lot over the years and I know for sure that when people suffer from various conditions for no logical reason, there is more likely than not an energetic carryover from the past that needs to be healed so it won't continue to wreak havoc on daily life.

From Victim to Victor

Hypnosis and guided imagery enable you to go back in time to the root cause of the issue, heal, and recognize the situation. Hypnotherapy transformed my life and has drastically improved the lives of thousands of people I've worked with over the years. I believe it can help you, too.

When upsetting things happen, there is a prevalent attitude in society that we are victims at the hands of fate and are at the mercy of our oppressors. I've lived a part of my life with that belief system myself, and I've found it simply does not work.

When you take a tangible action, even if it's only in your mind, to rid yourself of a perceived threat, you gain control over your future destiny and develop inner strength. The thoughts and images you form in your mind are real to you. Your brain has no way to differentiate between what is real in the three-dimensional universe versus what is imagined. By taking charge and directing what you think about by recreating traumatic events with a new-found sense of personal power, you can completely transform your life for the better.

From Karma to Dharma

It's important to understand what lessons you learned from various hardships, how you are applying those lessons to your current life situation, and how you can use that knowledge to improve your situation, or better yet, to help others. Once you find out why you chose to have a certain experience and can find the growth and the gift, then a real transformation can happen.

You see this all the time on the evening news. Recently there was a story about a little girl who had cancer. She had a tough fight and overcame her illness, so now she raises funding, supplies, and awareness to help other kids with cancer. She's taken her troubles and turned them into something of great service to her fellow human beings by mentally integrating her own journey to spiritu-ally move forward. The negative condition transformed and evolved into a vehi-cle to help others. She shifted her karma to dharma, or helpful energy, which is what I hope all of us can do as we journey on the path of healing.

When you can come to a place of being grateful for the tough times, knowing that energy can be used in the future to help others, then you've received the best gift of all. This is one of the most helpful aspects of my belief in reincarnation. Tragedy strikes all the time, but when you transform chal-lenging energy for a higher purpose, life becomes magical.

CHAPTER 2

· · · · · · · · ·

Introducing the RELIEF Method

THE GOAL OF PAST life regression is to relieve suffering by changing the way you view reality. RELIEF is an acronym I developed to describe the framework of the hypnotic process that allows you to journey back in time, rewrite your personal history, and live a more peaceful life in the present. RELIEF stands for the following:

- **Recognize:** Recognize the source of the anxiety or trauma and go back to the point of origin where the event first occurred.
- **Eliminate:** Eliminate the emotional charge by releasing fear or anxiety around the source event.
- **Lighten:** Lighten the frequency of the energy around a given event using healing and vibrational methods.
- **Integrate:** Integrate the new higher frequency energy into the physical, mental, and spiritual bodies by understanding the learning received from experiences.

- **Energize:** Energize internal thoughts, learnings, and holographic thoughtforms around the issue so they become incompatible with the lower frequencies of fear, stress, and anxiety.

- **Future:** Future progress into a scene in the current lifetime where the situation is completely resolved and healed. Bring that energy back to the present day and move on in life with a new perspective.

Let's explore each of these concepts in greater detail and I will explain why the process works so well for relieving anxiety, trauma, stress, and depression.

Recognize

*Recognize the source of the anxiety or trauma and go back
to the point of origin where the event first occurred.*

The only way to fully eliminate anxiety is to have the courage to discover and clear the true source event. A good analogy is a weed in your garden. You can repeatedly cut the weed off at the soil line, but unless you pull it out by the roots, it will continue to come back. The same principle applies to anxiety. Somewhere in the past there is a source event where the feelings and reactions from trauma began, and once that has been successfully identified and addressed at the point of origin, it is possible to create lasing change. Finding the root cause is not always as easy as it sounds. Sometimes you may think we know why you feel a certain way about an event, but under hypnosis, with the vast wellspring of your subconscious mind at your disposal, often surprising insights can arise. You will see several examples of that fact once we get into the case histories. Clients think a problem started in childhood, and then suddenly realize the real source happened hundreds of years ago.

The idea of going back and facing a fear sounds difficult, but since you are in the safe space of your mind and can view these events from a different perspective through the hypnotic process, tremendous healing can occur. During the regression I guide you to a safe place where you establish a protective shield, so you can safely travel to the point of origin, then by healing all events between then and now, you immediately shift and change. In sci-fi movies, a cliché scenario involves the paradox that if events were different and your grandfather was never born, then you would cease to exist. Likewise, when we go back to the past and either heal events by shifting them to something more positive, or eliminating them altogether, the source of anxiety is replaced by something more positive, all using the power of the mind.

Eliminate

Eliminate the emotional charge by releasing
fear or anxiety around the source event.

Once you recognize where an issue began, you begin the process of transformation by discovering and eliminating the emotional charge attached to the event. If you've experienced a painful relationship, for example—and of course we all have—sometimes a fight or disagreement leaves a bad taste in your mouth and creates a painful emotional charge. Without hypnosis or therapy, after some period of time goes by, you feel better because your subconscious tends to bury the pain so you can forget. That pain is still in the undercurrent of your mind though, so at some point down the road, those old feelings might reemerge. By eliminating the emotional charge attached to an event using the power of your imagination, you can spare yourself potentially years of emotional turmoil.

Another good example would be an electrical plug in your house. If one plug isn't working, you have to go out to the circuit breaker and reset the circuits by first turning off the switch and releasing the electrical charge. When our emotional circuits get bogged down with unpleasant emotions and conflict, eventually the physical body suffers. Have you ever had a string of Christmas lights stop working? That happens and you can't fix the problem until you identify the one or two tiny bulbs that are burned out. Once you replace that bulb or go to your circuit breaker and reset the circuits, you have changed the event and you've successfully reset the situation so the lights work again. Likewise, hypnosis helps you go in and find the tiny triggers that are causing disarray so you can clean them up and move forward again.

Not all past lives are challenging, of course, but typically with anxiety, depression, trauma, and the like, some negative trigger or event caused life to become difficult. Whatever the emotion you feel about the past—be it fear, anger, sadness, or even extreme joy—by rising above those feelings and gaining a new perspective, you can heal the emotional attachment and make lasting change.

When clients travel back to the source event, often I will guide them to see their own death or injuries, whether physical or emotional. Once they're observing the event, I have them notice an energetic cord between their physical body and the events or people from the past. Although we can't see them physically, these cords are quite real. Once the cord is cut, healing can begin. By taking ownership of their difficulties and choosing to eliminate challenges by facing them head-on, transformation can begin. Later in the book, you will have a chance to do some helpful cord-cutting processes.

Lighten

*Lighten the frequency of the energy around a given
event using healing and vibrational methods.*

Throughout my career, I have employed energy healing techniques in combination with past life regression. If there is heavy energy around a situation or event, by directing healing light to that area and raising the lower frequencies to higher ones, unwanted influences are no longer compatible with the new higher vibrations and these disturbances disappear.

You've likely heard the saying *thoughts are things,* and that is very true. There is an energetic component to memory, meaning there is an actual unseen yet nevertheless real energy that surrounds all our memories, whether they are from this life or the past. When I guide you into your past lives and you recall an event verbally, in order to completely transform the situation, you must also address the energetic thoughtform, as I call it, around that past life. A thought-form is like a ball of energy that represents the memory. For example, if I ask you to think of a toy you had as a child and hold it in your mind, you may imagine it just out in front of your face. You might see how it looked; recall the texture and feeling you had about the toy. Likewise, memories from past lives can also be recalled and occupy physical space unseen by the naked eye. These unseen energy fields must be shifted for the situation to be completely healed.

A good example is a rainy day. Let's say clouds are covering the skies and it's pouring outside. Then the winds of change arrive, blowing the clouds out of the way, dispersing the darkness so the sunshine comes through. Lightening the event is very similar, although it's all done on an energetic level in your mind. The process is very effective for changing the nature of an unpleasant situation.

Integrate

Integrate the new higher frequency energy into the physical, mental, and spiritual bodies by understanding the learning received from experiences.

When we incarnate, we are spiritual beings who choose to experience this physical world in order to grow and learn. As such, we can energetically shift our frequencies by lightening events, which is good to do, but we must also intellectually understand why certain things happened, and what our souls learned through the process. Recognizing and acknowledging our lessons is necessary for soul growth.

Our bodies occupy physical space, and yet we actually are all energy. Our energy field is capable of expanding up to thirty feet around our physical bodies. When I teach energy healing, I break the layers of this infinite, expanding field into three parts: physical, mental, and spiritual. Different memories and blockages get stuck in these unseen fields and will eventually wreak havoc on us if they are not cleared out. Over the years I've learned that it's not enough to talk through past life regressions. While it's wonderful to discuss past lives so we can intellectually come to terms with various aspects of our soul's development, once that's done, we must experience a corresponding energetic shift by raising the vibrations of the unseen aspects of the corresponding memory in order for change to last.

Aside from shifting the thoughtforms, or energetic component, around events, the other way energy shifts to higher frequencies is by determining what the soul learned from past events and how those situations are affecting you in the now. Life can be challenging. We all know that, and yet even the most difficult situations can foster soul growth; knowing that things really do happen for a reason helps us accept and integrate those challenges into our being so we can benefit from them. Karma implies the sum of past events, and when we can use our past to benefit our soul's learning and help others, we shift karma into dharma, or helpful energy. The realization of how we benefit from even the most painful situations instantly raises the frequency of the energy and creates lasting change.

Energize

*Energize internal thoughts and learnings and holographic
thoughtforms around the issue so they become incompatible
with the lower frequencies of fear, stress, and anxiety.*

You may have heard the old saying *perception is reality.* Well, it's true. We talked about adding light to the situation. Once that's done, the frequency and vibration of that energy is raised even further within the light bodies.

Within your physical shell, you have an infinite ball of light that is your spirit or soul. In healing work, different layers of this light body relate to issues of the physical body, mind, and spirit. When you address your learnings and raise the frequencies of this light so that energetic blockages and karma are cleared from the body, mind, and spirit, lasting change is achieved. Depression, trauma, and anxiety can no longer exist in the newly created environment of healing.

Throughout the RELIEF Method, work is done to energize your field, so this step further shifts the energy field in support of new thoughts, learning, and decisions.

Future

*Journey into a future event in the current lifetime where the situation is
completely resolved and healed. Bring that new energy back to the present day
and move forward in life toward the future with the desired outcome in mind.*

To ensure you've made the desired change, the best way to test the change is to journey into the future in your current lifetime so you can see, feel, and experience yourself enjoying life and experience newfound joy while realizing that, without a doubt, your difficulty is a thing of the past. All time is now, which is why you can actually travel out into your current life future to see the things you truly want in life working out for you.

I see this step as a sort of reverse engineering for the soul. Let's say, for example, we wanted to know how to build a sports car and understand all the inner workings of a car. If possible, it would be easier to build the car if we could take apart an existing one and then figure out how it works. Your soul journey can be the same. Because all things are possible, you can simply go to a wonderful event in your current life future and see how you created the desired outcome. By traveling out to a future memory in your current life where you are happy, healthy, and living your ideal life, your soul can easily discover the exact steps you took to create that change, so when your journey is over, you can move in that direction and generate greater joy in your life.

The information received from your future can be incredibly specific and detailed. If you make note of the ideal steps and leave the regression with a commitment to follow your own advice, incredibly positive change will occur. You have all the power and resources within, and this step solidifies your ability to create the life you truly want to live and invest your past history into making life all the better for yourself, those around you, and the world at large. The future, paradoxically, is critical to the regression because otherwise, why would we bother to seek answers if we cannot receive a tangible benefit? Of course, it's interesting to know who you were in the past, but the real gift is using the information now to make the most out of your current life.

Example of the RELIEF Method in Action

In part two, you'll read several interesting case histories of clients who benefited from the RELIEF Method. Because I won't be outlining the steps throughout those studies, in the following example, I will share Rachel's story to show you exactly how the RELIEF Method works. Please keep in mind that all client names and details are disguised to protect privacy. Here's what happened.

Recognition of the Source Event

Rachel had a terrible fear of the dark she couldn't resolve after years of traditional therapy. During her regression, she successfully accessed the source event when she traveled to her life in 1700s rural America and experienced herself tumbling down a dark flight of stairs to her death.

Eliminate the Emotional Charge

To release the emotional charge, in this case *fear*, surrounding her accident, I asked Rachel to lift up out of her past life and cut an energetic cord with the accident victim. In the next section, you'll see plenty of examples of acknowl-edging, then disconnecting from, beams of light that exist between clients and unwanted conditions. In part three, you'll experience this process yourself.

Lighten the Situation

Once Rachel disconnected from her former self, I sent energy to help her heal from the shock. During this time, we discussed the fact that what had happened then had nothing to do with her current life. I also had her imag-ine a bright healing light banishing the darkness she so feared, and we talked through this until she reported feeling better.

Integrate

Hearing that the events from her deep past did not need to affect her in the now is all well and good, but at some point, Rachel had to process that infor-mation and come to terms with the fact that she no longer needed to fear the dark. Integration means that the mental comprehension must transform into actual experience. I spoke to Rachel about feeling safe, and we talked through the fact that her past no longer needed to affect her current life. While she processed the information, I continued to work on her energetically until she shifted.

Energize

The energizing step involved Rachel further imagining herself surrounded by healing light so that every single cell in her body relaxed and disconnected from her fear. I relied on Rachel's feedback and waited until she verbally told me she felt better.

Future

The only way I know for sure my clients have succeeded in making the desired change is to guide them into their future. I asked Rachel to go to a moment in her current life where she could see and experience herself healed from her fear of the dark. Rachel accessed a future memory where she was alone in the dark while feeling completely unafraid. That's when I knew the process was complete. The future component is critical for the RELIEF Method to work because clients must believe they have actually changed by experiencing a new outcome. That's what happened for Rachel, and that's what can happen for you too.

Summing Up

If you believe in what you experience and move forward after the session as if your vision is true, then miracles can happen. In order to fully achieve lasting change, you must release the past trauma, get the lessons, and then go out into the future where you can see yourself living a better life, having completely overcome the situation causing your anxiety. This is powerful. One of the biggest gifts of the regression process is the fact that while you're in the hypnotic state, you can consciously recall all the details that go on during a session. By taking notes afterwards, you will easily recall the soul lessons and can develop a written action plan of how you will proceed to create the life you want using the detailed information you uncovered during your session. In part three of the book, I will guide you step-by-step through the journaling process to help you get the most out of your sessions. Once you know RELIEF is in sight and can actually feel and experience those results and the benefits of your new belief in your own healing, the sky's the limit on what you can accomplish. Once you return from your regression and understand the steps you can take to create a more empowered future in your current lifetime, moving forward courageously and following your plan is the key to success.

PART TWO

· · · · ·

Case Studies

IF YOU'RE ALIVE ON our planet, then at some point you've experienced anxiety and fear. That's simply part of being human. Under normal circumstances, everyone can handle a little stress once in a while, but when anxiety becomes extreme, overly traumatic, or constant, things can get out of hand and life becomes quite difficult.

According to Buddhist philosophy, all beings suffer. Some people's struggles are more visible, such as a physical challenge, while others suffer silently. Anxiety, trauma, and depression are among these silent sufferings sadly experienced by too many people today. The good news is that several anxiety disorders are now fully recognized by the American Psychiatric Association, so the stigmas once associated with such diagnoses have been lessened.

With so many people suffering from anxiety these days, I know for a fact that many cope with these issues without seeking any help at all. Maybe that's you. My wish is that through hearing about the journeys of other people, you may find a sense that you are not alone, and like the people in the examples you're about to read, you can experience a brighter tomorrow.

Next, I will share some fascinating case histories so you can see how regular people learned to view the world through different lenses by rewriting their life stories, relieving some of their silent suffering and healing through past life regression. As a reminder, I've changed all names and omitted personal details to protect privacy.

In part three, I will offer several of the exercises you can try yourself to help you relieve suffering as well. For now, let's take a look at the case studies.

CHAPTER 3

Fear & Phobias

IT'S SAFE TO SAY that everybody alive is afraid of something. You may be afraid of flying, or deep water, or spiders. Even Indiana Jones was deathly afraid of snakes, and there's nothing wrong with that. In fact, some fears are totally justified and are genetically built into your DNA to keep you safe. But when fears get out of hand, they can keep you from living a full life.

Phobia

General fear can become debilitating and intensify into a phobia, which is defined by the American Psychiatric Association's *Diagnostic and Statistical Manual of Mental Disorders* (DSM-5) as "individuals who suffer from intense fear or anxiety when exposed to specific objects or situations."

I know from firsthand experience that most people have something from their past that causes extreme distress or fear. I developed a dog phobia after being attacked at the age of four. My journey to relief from what had become a lifelong challenge was exactly that—a journey. Relief didn't happen overnight, but with time and after completely reframing my thinking and having a past life regression, I improved. The same can happen for you.

You may have experienced something traumatic that happened to you at a tender age. When you're a child, you're wide open to everything, which is why such incidents can wreak havoc on future behavior. Regressing back to those sources of trauma, even when they happened in your current life, can prove quite beneficial when you're ready.

Over the years, I've encountered several clients who used past life regression to overcome their phobias. Of course, it's always possible that the source of fear originated in current life events, such as my experience with the dog attack. And yet our souls are complex, so oftentimes a deeper healing is necessary, as in the following case studies of people who successfully overcame their fears.

Carol Feared Tunnels for No Reason

In the very first part of the book, I briefly mentioned Carol, who feared traveling through tunnels in either her car or on trains. When she had her first past life regression, Carol initially said she didn't see a thing, then later admitted that a tiny vision came through about her being in a dark place when everything turned black. That happens quite often. People may or may not get anything when they first try to do a past life regression. Hypnotic work is like exercising a muscle at the gym. The more you do it, the easier it gets. Later in the book I will give you a series of exercises to do at home that are designed to build up your muscles and help you get more insights and healing over time.

It's important to know that it is okay if you don't get anything the very first time you try regression. That happens for a reason. Unfortunately, sometimes when this happens, a client might drop their inquiry altogether and not bother getting to the bottom of the root cause because they falsely believe they cannot be hypnotized, or they can't access past lives, or they don't have any past lives. I've found that's not true. They likely have past lives, but they're not ready to access the information. If the memories were meant to come up, they would. By continuing to try, over time, when one is ready, incredible healing can result.

That's exactly what happened to me. During my first past life regression, I only saw a nanosecond of a flash of some cowboy boots with no explanation and no other insights at all. I dropped the ball on trying regression and several years passed before I went back to try again. To my surprise, on my second attempt, I received insight into the cowboy boots I'd seen years earlier. As it turned out, those boots were the key to a major life issue. After nine long years, I still struggled with unresolved grief over the death of my dear friend who had died in the hiking accident. I discovered he was my wife in a prior life and while I was out, my wife and children had been brutally murdered by bandits. Those boots I had seen in my vision years earlier were my boots and the second time I went to that exact life, more details emerged. I saw inside my former home and received answers to help heal my grief. How I wish I had gone in for that second regression sooner! I could have spared myself years of misery. Then again, I've always believed everything happens as it should, in its own time. Unfortunately, God's time, so to speak, often takes far longer than what we'd like.

Therefore, I was incredibly pleased when Carol came back to see me again so soon. Once she admitted to seeing something, that meant her soul and Higher Self were ready to heal. Remember, your subconscious is always going to keep you safe, so it's important to be gentle with yourself and allow your memories and healing to unfold in their own time, which is exactly what happened with Carol. We met for a second regression, and during the time in between, she mentioned another new experience she had after her regression:

"Ever since we first met, even though I didn't see much, I started having a lot of dreams. I can't tell you what they were about because I'd remember them the second I woke up and by the time I got out of bed, they'd be gone. I guess I should have written them down, but oh well. Even though I can't remember, I know they had to do with the tunnels. It's just a feeling I have. I think I've been working things out in my mind while I sleep, if that makes any sense. Sounds crazy, I know."

Carol's description sounded perfectly normal to me. Your subconscious mind works out details for you while you sleep, better preparing you to handle new information in the waking three-dimensional world. When she went on the journey again, following the steps of the regression, that time the insights opened up and Carol received relevant answers:

Shelley Kaehr (SK): Surrounded by healing, protective light, safe and secure, go back to the source event of your fear of tunnels and be there now. Notice what's happening. Where are you?

Carol: South America.

SK: What year is this?

Carol: (hesitating) 1800s? I'm not sure.

SK: Very good. What's happening in South America in the 1800s?

Carol: I am very poor. We're in the mountains.

SK: Are you a man or woman?

Carol: Woman.

SK: Are you alone or with other people?

Carol: I am with lots of people from my village. We're walking down a path through the forest.

SK: As you experience the energy of the people from the village, is there anyone there you recognize from your current life, yes or no?

Carol: No.

SK: Fast forward from that moment and see where you go. Remember you are still surrounded by a protective light so that only that which is of your highest good can come through. Notice what happens next.

Carol: We're going up to a cave. There's something inside we need. The men are telling us to wait while they go farther back inside. They leave and I am waiting with a couple other women and some little children. It is starting to rain and it is very cold so we go inside to get out of the cold and ... oh!

SK: What's happening?

Carol: I hear a rumble.

SK: Thunder?

Carol: No, it's from deeper inside the cave. We make a mistake and start running toward the noise, further into the cave. We want to check on the others.

SK: Surrounded by light, fast forward to the next most significant event. Be there now.

Carol: The cave collapsed! Dirt and rocks are falling everywhere. We can't get out! Everyone else who is further inside is crushed. (emotional) It's awful.

SK: Go to the last day of your life, be there now, notice how you pass into spirit.

Carol: I am hit on the head. I black out and die of suffocation. Other than the fear, though, I didn't suffer. Others had it much worse.

SK: Very good. Float up, up, up, into that peaceful space in between lives. Be there now. Safe and secure. Imagine your guide can send a healing light down over those events, healing and calming, bringing peace to that cave. Let me know when it feels better.

Carol: (after a few minutes) Yes.

SK: What lessons did you learn in that life in South America?

Carol: Loyalty at all costs. If we had not been as loyal, we would have run out of the cave instead of inside and we would have lived, but it would have been a struggle to survive without the men around to help with hunting and keeping us safe.

SK: Do you regret that?

Carol: No.

SK: How does that life relate to what you're doing in your current life?

Carol: I've had issues at work, as you know, and I think I'm being way too loyal to people who don't deserve it. I'm not in a life-or-death situation anymore and, in this life, in order to save myself, I need to get out while I can.

In our earlier session when Carol claimed she didn't see any past lives, she initially came to see me not only to discover the source of her fear of tunnels but to discuss her dismay at working for a highly unethical manager who did several things that went against her values. She felt trapped into staying, fearing she might not get another position.

SK: How does this situation in the cave relate to your fear of tunnels?

Carol: I always thought I feared tunnels because I never really go into the mountains at all in this lifetime. I told my husband I do not camp, I will not go out into any of those kinds of places, so once in a while, he takes our kids hiking while I stay home. The tunnels remind me of the caves for some reason, but I can see now I have no real reason to be afraid of tunnels.

SK: You are certain that this life in South America is the true source event of your fear of tunnels in your current lifetime?

Carol: Oh yes, definitely.

SK: Very good. Now travel to the future in your current life, to an event where you are happy, healthy, and easily able to drive a car through a tunnel. Be there now, notice what's happening.

Carol: It's several years from now. I am in the car with my husband and we're driving on a winding road in some mountains.

SK: How do you feel?

Carol: Great, actually. I have never been anywhere like this with him before. Our kids are staying with my parents and it feels fun, like we're getting away, doing something for ourselves for a change.

SK: Good job. Notice what happens next.

Carol: There is a tunnel on the road. I see the car driving toward it and I am not shaking or upset. I feel good.

SK: Do you go through the tunnel?

Carol: Yes.

SK: Good job. Go ahead and do that now, let me know what happens as you move through the tunnel to the other side.

Carol: The car is getting closer, but I feel okay. I can see there is a tile roof and walls on this one and there are a few lights on so it's not completely dark. We are moving inside and driving through. A car passes us and has its headlights on. I feel really good actually. I'm surprised. Now we're already on the other side. It didn't take long at all, and oh! It's so beautiful over here! We've crossed into a green valley with lots of tiny cabins and beautiful trees!

SK: How do you feel now?

Carol: Kind of regretful that I didn't get over my fear a long time ago. I can see now that there are a lot of neat places I missed because I was too scared to go anywhere. Now I can look forward to doing more in the future, though.

SK: And from that future event in the mountains, imagine you can remember back to your earlier life and notice if you still work in the same place or not.

Carol: Oh no, not at all. I quit there immediately after our session.

SK: Very good, and when you quit, what happened? Imagine you know because you are in the future now and these things have already happened.

Carol: I went in, shortly after the session, actually, and I gave my two weeks' notice. I did not have another job at the time, but I talked to some neighbors and one of them knew someone who hired me with no problem. I didn't have to say anything against my employer either, which was good. I told the new manager that I needed better hours and more pay, and I got both.

SK: How do you feel in this future event, knowing you work in a new place you enjoy and can see the world with greater ease, traveling through tunnels to new places?

Carol: Life is good. Everything's better now.

Even though Carol regretted not addressing her phobia sooner, her personal insights were revealed exactly when Carol was ready to receive them, and she happily moved forward with her life and took charge of her situation by empowering herself to find a new job with people who shared her values. We spoke some time after our session, and I was thrilled to hear Carol followed through on our session and made changes, although they were not exactly how she had foreseen them.

"I did quit that other company, although I didn't just walk out. I couldn't do that in my real life because I needed the money too much. I asked some neighbors if they knew anyone who was hiring and one of them had a friend who referred me to my current job. Several months after our session, I put in my two weeks' notice and changed jobs. I still haven't had a chance to go through any tunnels yet though, so I'm not sure how that's gonna work, but based on my new job and how much happier I am, I feel like good things are coming."

While things did not materialize exactly the way she had seen, Carol managed to find greater happiness after she integrated her new insights, and that's all that matters. Moving forward on the path of life, doing our best, one step at a time, is all any of us can be expected to do.

A Past Life Car Accident Made Ashley Antsy

On the subject of tunnels, I also worked with Ashley, whom I met during one of my group regression classes. She mentioned being deathly afraid to drive in stormy or inclement weather.

Group settings can be helpful for bringing up fragments of issues that need deeper healing, which is what happened to Ashley. During our group session, she experienced the following:

"I saw a flash of a car accident on a mountain pass sometime in the 1950s, and I feel like I need to come in and do a full regression to get to the bottom of this, because I first started having anxiety in my car after my boyfriend, who is now my husband, tried taking me up to Colorado for a ski vacation. I cried and practically came unglued on the roads there. They were icy and slick, and I about made myself sick. I know he thought I was nuts, and I'm surprised he married me after that but he did. Only now, I tell him I won't go skiing ever again, because even if we fly into Denver, for example, we'd still have to drive on those roads. I won't do it. I just can't, and I've gotten so bad that I won't even leave my house when it rains. I know he wishes I'd drop it, though. We both do like to ski."

During our private past life regression, Ashley accessed the source of her anxiety on the first try:

SK: Where are you and what's happening?

Ashley: Somewhere in Europe in the early 1950s. I'm a passenger in a car, the roads are slick with a rainy, icy mix and we're about to go into a tunnel. There's a super slippery part of the road inside the tunnel and our car swerves into the other lane, hitting an oncoming truck. We are both killed at the scene.

SK: Go ahead and leave that body, and that life, floating into the peaceful space in between lives. Allow a healing light to move down over those events in the tunnel, melting away all fears and trauma. What lessons did you learn in that life in the 1950s?

Ashley: Be cautious.

SK: How is that affecting you now?

Ashley: I've taken it too far. Yes, you need to be careful, but not at the expense of enjoying life. We're all going to die and there's nothing we can do about it. Whether I liked it or not, my time was up on that road. If it's not your time, you aren't going. Death is nothing to fear. I need to enjoy.

SK: Travel out into your current life, to a time when the weather is bad and you are driving. Imagine easily driving without fear. What year is it?

Ashley: It's this winter. The roads are slick. It's raining; not snowing yet. I'm cooking dinner and I forgot something. I call my husband because I want him to pick it up on the way home from work, but he's not answering his cell, so I drive out into the rain.

SK: How do you feel?

Ashley: Good, actually. I drive to the store, walk inside, get what I need, and get home safely.

SK: Great!

Ashley proved that with a few new insights, life can begin anew by changing thought patterns. I ran into her some time later and she had made major changes since her session.

"I still try to avoid bad weather when I can, but I'm able to live more freely than before. I won't stay home just because of rain. I feel so much better and my life isn't limited like it was before the session. I'm truly at peace now."

Achieving the confidence to go out and enjoy life is a great goal for anyone having a past life regression. I was incredibly proud of Ashley for embracing her own inner wisdom and using the experience as a growth opportunity. People are often way too hard on themselves. Yes, we all make mistakes and potentially lose valuable time, but once change is made and improvements happen, then you should congratulate yourself for changing and not lament wasted opportunity. Life is a learning ground and as long as you learn and grow, that's all you can expect of yourself. Ashley did a wonderful job with expanding her life in light of her new insights about her soul journey.

Wasps & Bees Loved Fearful Sarah

Lots of people are afraid of bees for good reason. Bee stings can kill some people who have harsh allergic reactions. I met Sarah, a girl in her early twenties, at an outdoor metaphysical event and couldn't help noticing wasps and bees swarming around her, causing her extreme distress.

"Have you ever been stung?" I asked her.

"No, but I have a phobia of bees. They won't stop bothering me!"

My ears perked up when she actually used the term *phobia* to describe her fear. The Law of Attraction says the more you pay attention to things, whether they are good or bad, the more they manifest. So suffice it to say, I was beyond curious to see why the insects were so attracted to her. We did a short healing session during the fair. I sent her some energy, balancing her chakra centers while I guided Sarah back to the source of her relationship with wasps and bees.

SK: Be there now and notice the first time you encountered wasps or bees, the time that is most affecting you now. What year is this and where are you? Notice the first thing that comes to your mind.

Sarah: 1700s. Holland.

SK: What's happening?

Sarah: I am working outside around the flowers. The bees are everywhere. I can't get away from them.

SK: How old are you?

Sarah: I am a girl there, too, not very old—ten, maybe? I have a little sister and the bees are swarming and stinging her. She gets sick and dies.

SK: How is this affecting you in your current life?

Sarah: I am afraid that will happen to me.

SK: Imagine you can talk to the bees that are here today and in your current life. Take your time and tell them that you do not wish to see them anymore. Notice there is an energetic cord between you and these bees. When I count down from three, we will cut the cord, freeing you from the bees. Three, two, one, cutting that cord. A gorgeous healing light is surrounding you now, creating a protective shell, healing you from the past and keeping the bees away from your energy field. Let me know when this is better.

Sarah: Yes, it feels better.

SK: What about the wasps? Why are they around? Go to the source event of your troubles and be there now.

Sarah: There is nothing to see. The only reason they bother me is because I am afraid of the bees.

SK: So you don't have any past lives with wasps that need healing?

Sarah: No.

SK: Are you ready to release your connection to the wasps?

Sarah: Yes.

SK: When are you ready to do that?

Sarah: Now.

SK: Good. Go ahead and cut the cords, bringing a healing light down from above, imagine it is totally releasing you from your fear and let me know when this feels healed and resolved.

Sarah: (in a moment) Yes, it's much better.

When Sarah returned from the short journey, she went around the fair and toward the end of the day, stopped back by my booth.

"I can't believe it," she said. "The bees haven't come near me ever since we did our session."

I was thrilled, to say the least. Sarah is a wonderful example of the fact that changes can be made that have an immediate impact on your life. That's one of the main reasons I became a hypnotherapist in the first place. The human mind is so powerful that with the proper instructions, you can turn everything around in an instant. And, of course, this case history left me reaffirming the fact that there's something to that Law of Attraction stuff after all. Change the way you view things inside, and your whole world transforms on the outside. Simple!

Jenny Wouldn't Leave Home to Search for Work

If you're afraid of venturing out in public, you may be agoraphobic, officially defined by the DSM-5 as a "diagnosis assigned to individuals who have a disproportionate fear of public places, perceiving such environments as too open, crowded, or dangerous."

With all the bad news in the media these days, I wouldn't be surprised if anyone hesitated to venture into public places or talked themselves out of leaving home. At times, these feelings are caused not by modern disasters at all, but by events that occurred long, long ago. That's exactly what happened with Jenny, who had a session with me shortly after being laid off from her job.

A distraught Jenny had never been let go or fired in her entire life and felt depressed beyond belief. Fortunately, her husband had a good job, yet her anxiety persisted. What made matters worse was an unexplainable internal conflict that she could not resolve.

"I know I need to get out there and look for work but something's stopping me. When I think about having to go to interviews or job fairs, a deeprooted fear comes over me."

We did a regression to find the source event.

SK: Be there now. What's happening? Where are you?

Jenny: It's sometime in the 1930s on the East Coast, although I'm not sure exactly where I am, other than I see myself standing in a long line, holding a little girl's hand. We're moving slowly and we're so hungry. After a time, I notice we've managed to make our way up toward the front of the line, and I can see what's there. Bread and a thin cup of broth, if you could even call it that. It's lukewarm and doesn't have a lot in it in terms of nutrition. This is a bread line. (She begins to cry.) We're too poor to help ourselves and there are no jobs.

SK: Fast forward through this scene and notice what happens next.

Jenny: I get the broth for me and my little girl, and we have to drink it there so we can give the cup back for someone else to use it. There's no way to wash dishes, nothing is clean. It's so unsanitary. It tastes horrible, actually, but it's filling in the aching space in my stomach. My little girl is so weak, she can barely walk, but she looks better now.

We're leaving the line with a loaf of bread to take home. That will get us through the next day. I walk away from the crowd and we're crossing a street, going into an alley in between two large brick buildings. A man jumps out at us. He pulls a knife and stabs me right in the stomach. I'm falling in the alley, bleeding to death, but I can only think about my little girl. I tell her to run, which she does, and the man gets away with the bread. As far as I know, he did not hurt my little girl, but I'm lying there panicked because I can't be there for her anymore. I don't want to die! Not today! Not like this! Who's gonna watch her? How will she survive?

Still crying, she lifted up into the blissful space in between lives.

SK: What lessons did you learn and how is this affecting you now?

Jenny: I'm about the same age now as I was when I died in my last life. I'm not destitute like I was then, so there's no need to worry. I can see my little girl grew up in that life and became strong. I learned that no matter how much you want to live, if it's your time to go, you're going. My life now is perfect in comparison. I have to brave the job market and I know things won't ever be that bad again. If I don't get a job, I won't die. I have to be open to going out there and trying.

The next time I heard from her, she had a new job. She wasn't making quite as much as before, but she was happy and that's all that mattered. Curious about how difficult it might have been to initially push through the fear and put herself out there, I asked her about that when we spoke.

"It wasn't easy at first. I had to do a lot of talking to myself about the fact that I am okay now and that even if nobody hires me, I'd live. I put things into proper perspective. As it turned out, the first company I interviewed with hired me, and I've enjoyed it so far."

Even if you receive insights after a past life regression or any other healing or therapy you try, at some point, you still have to take action and move forward with confidence in order for the healing and resolution to occur. Jenny did an amazing job of acknowledging her fears and going out there anyway, and that's what we all must do in order to live fulfilling lives.

Melody Feared the Office

When Melody came to see me, she struggled with several issues, including the fact that she panicked every time she had to go into the office. She tele-commuted most of the time and seemed fine on the outside, but internally she suffered. When I questioned Melody more specifically about what caused these feelings, I asked if she had either a difficult boss or coworkers.

"That's the problem," she explained. "There is no problem. *I'm* the prob-lem. My boss is super nice. I don't know the people in the office very well because I don't go in, but when I do, they've always been nice. There's some-thing more that I'm not getting."

We traveled into Melody's past and discovered the source event in her childhood.

SK: How old are you?

Melody: Five.

SK: What's happening?

Melody: My stepfather is yelling at me. My real dad died when I was a baby and my mom married a monster. They're divorced now. He was a ver-bally abusive control freak who always shouted at both of us.

SK: Did he hurt you?

Melody: Not physically, no, but I can see his face now. I hadn't thought about him in years, but my boss has similar features.

I attempted to have her cut the cords with her stepfather, but when I asked her to do so, she surprised me.

Melody: I can't.

SK: Why not?

Melody: I don't know.

SK: Go back to the source event, the first time you ever encountered the soul whom you've known as your stepfather. Be there now. Where are you?

Melody: This seems strange, but I want to say Byzantine Empire. (chuckling) I'm not even sure what that means.

SK: Good job. So, what's happening in the Byzantine Empire?

Melody: I'm poor, struggling. There's fighting all around, smoke and darkness, diseases. It's really bad.

SK: Look around. Notice if there are other people with you, and if so, what are they doing?

Melody: We're all poor, struggling to find food. I stole some bread because I had to, and now I'm being punished and beaten.

SK: As you experience the energy of the people around you, is there anybody you know from your current life?

Melody: It's him. My stepfather. He's beating me and arresting me for stealing. He's some kind of soldier and has no empathy for any of us.

SK: Very good. Fast forward to the last day of your life in the Byzantine Empire and be there now. Notice how it is as you pass into spirit.

Melody: I'm taken away with several beggars. I don't know what they expect us to do. We're starving to death. They put us in a cell with no food and I die before I can be executed.

SK: Float up and out of that body, into the peaceful space in between lives. Be there now. Safe and secure, invite the soldier who arrested you to come forward and imagine he can apologize to you for what he did.

Melody: He won't. He says he did his job.

SK: Good, then imagine that even if he won't apologize, you can forgive him anyway. Can you do that?

Melody: I think so.

SK: Bring a healing light over you both and notice an energetic cord between you. When I count down from three, we will cut that cord. Three, two, one, cut. Let me know when it feels better.

Melody: (after a few moments) Yes.

SK: Now bring your stepfather out. Imagine this is his Higher Self, his soul, talking to your soul. What lessons are the two of you learning about together?

Melody: Tolerance, although he never learned.

SK: Can his Higher Self apologize to you?

Melody: No.

SK: Would you be willing to forgive him his transgressions anyway, so you can move on?

Melody: I can forgive, but I won't ever forget.

SK: Fair enough. Notice that energetic cord between you? This represents all the cruel behavior he directed toward you. When I count to three, we will cut that cord and you will release him because you are too strong to be affected by this any longer—one, two, three, cutting the cord. Let me know when this feels better.

Melody: (after a moment) Okay, it's better.

SK: Nice. So, tell me, how is this situation with your stepfather affecting your feelings about going into the office in your current life?

Melody: My boss looks like him, which is what bothered me. I guess I needed this session because I never realized how much my stepfather affected me until now.

SK: Good job. Go ahead and float away from your stepfather and out into your future to a moment when you decide to drive to your office to work. Imagine you notice how happily you go inside, greet your boss and coworkers, and go about your day. Let me know what's happening.

Melody: It's a week from now. My boss had been out at a conference but he's back now. I didn't have to go in, but I found out he would be in so I made a point of driving to work.

SK: How do you feel?

Melody: It's like night and day. So much better.

SK: How do you feel with your coworkers?

Melody: I'm smiling more, asking them how they're doing, and they're asking me the same. They're really nice people when I take the time to get to know them better.

SK: Very good. Now go to your boss and notice how you interact with him.

Melody: I go up to say good morning to him and he smiles and says hello.

SK: Nice! Look at your boss. How do you feel about him in general?

Melody: I'm over seeing him as someone who reminds me of my step-father. He's just my boss. He's a good person. Treats everyone with respect.

SK: Great! Imagine you can fast forward in time and notice how this new feeling about your work is affecting your office environment and your relationship with your boss and coworkers now that you've changed.

Melody: He's reacting better to me now because I'm actually approaching him. I never realized how much I avoided him before, but I'm so much better now. I'm happier at my job. I'm getting to be friends with some of the people at work. We go to lunch together and I drive into the office more so I am part of the team.

I caught up with Melody via email about a month after our session to find out how things in the real world were going, and she reported that she had made a conscious effort to go into the office once a week whether she had to or not, and she formed new friendships and a better working relationship with her boss, who actually gave her new, more complex assignments to tackle. Overall, she felt happier and relieved.

Summing Up

Sometimes things we fear in our minds turn out to be nothing in the real world, especially once a healing occurs. Life gets better in a moment's notice. Each of the clients you read about demonstrated that when you change the interior thoughts of how you project onto the world around you, everything changes.

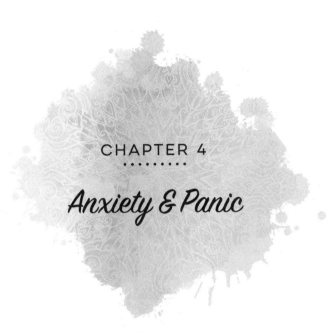

CHAPTER 4

Anxiety & Panic

IN THIS CHAPTER, WE will explore past life case studies from people who experienced often-debilitating anxiety and panic, only to find relief from their deep-rooted past rather than from anything in their current lives.

Anxiety

According to the DSM-5, some of the many symptoms of generalized anxiety include "excessive anxiety and worry (apprehensive expectation), occurring more days than not for at least six months, about a number of events (such as work or school performance)."

While the clients you're about to read about did not necessarily qualify for a clinical diagnosis, they certainly experienced instances of anxiety, sometimes causing panic attacks or similar symptoms.

Mary Released Chronic Anxiety

Mary suffered from deep-rooted issues with anxiety throughout her life. She tried different medications and when none worked to her satisfaction, she chose a spiritual path of meditation and mindfulness to try to alleviate her stress. Everything went smoothly for her for years, until life issues caused her anxiety to rear its ugly head again, worse than ever.

"I've been doing so well for so long," she told me, "but ever since my husband and I decided to call it quits and file for divorce, I've been a nervous wreck. I stayed home to raise my daughter and I own a small business that doesn't bring in nearly enough money to make ends meet. Now I'm going to have to move and somehow find a job."

We did quite a bit of forgiveness and healing work around her divorce as she gratefully acknowledged the gifts her marriage had given her, but knew she had to move on. Then, surprisingly, when I asked her to travel to the source of her anxiety, she soon realized she experienced these exact feelings before in her past life.

> *SK:* What year is this and what's happening?
>
> *Mary:* I'm on a beach wearing a swimsuit. It's 1932 and my swimsuit is white with puffy long sleeves and knee-length bloomers with ruffles. I'm barefoot. I'm with two young girls who are my friends from school. I'm 16 years old. I see a boardwalk off in the distance, with carnival rides and music playing. I'm so happy. I feel that my family is privileged with money.
>
> *Mary:* Very good. Go ahead now and fast forward to the next most significant event in the 1930s. Be there now. Where are you? What's happening?
>
> *Mary:* Now it's two years later, my father dies from cancer, and I have to go to work to support myself. I'm really scared and I don't know how I'll make it.
>
> *SK:* Good job. Is there anything about that situation that reminds you of your current life, yes or no?
>
> *Mary:* Oh yes, it's just the same, only different. I had a life of abundance until all of a sudden, I had the rug pulled out from under me, and now I'm on my own.
>
> *SK:* Notice the energy of the father in that lifetime. Is he anyone you know in your current life?
>
> *Mary:* Oh my gosh! It's him! My soon-to-be ex! He's so much older than I am in that life, and he's older than me in this life too.

SK: What lessons did the two of you come together to learn?

Mary: We support each other, we're good friends, and think the same on a lot of levels. The problem is that we're not meant to be together forever. We're together for a reason and for a shorter period of time. It's not meant to last. That's part of my learning. I must learn how to stand up on my own two feet. He's helping me do that by forcing me out.

SK: Great! Travel out further into your life in the 1930s and notice what happened after your father passed away.

Mary: I had a very average existence after that. I always cherished my younger life and my teenage years. I missed that life! Then again, I had everything I needed. I learned that you don't need all that wealth to be happy.

SK: And were you happy in that life?

Mary: I was, yes.

SK: Travel out beyond today and go into a moment in your current-life future where you are happy, healthy, through with your divorce, and successfully standing on your own. Be there now. Notice what's happening.

Mary: It's a few years from now. I live in my other house south of here and I love it. The scenery is so much prettier than where I lived when I was married. I went back to school about five years ago, so now I'm actually using my degree. I'm a teacher, I make really good money, and I live in my house, which is paid for. I have a really nice life, and what's better is I'm so much happier on my own. My ex and I are still great friends, but we didn't need to be together anymore. He's doing well and everything worked out.

Incredibly, the things Mary foresaw in her future came true. She's one of the best examples of someone who went into her empowered future and actually took the steps to move forward into her happier, fuller life. I am quite proud of her. She is doing wonderful these days.

This level of success can happen for you too! Later in the book in the guided journeys section, you will have opportunities to travel into your future and discover the best plans for a happy life and learn the steps you will take to move forward in the direction of your highest potential. Using hypnosis, you will use guided visualizations and the power of your imagination to go see your own future. It's truly empowering to see your own highest potential and then move forward into the life you've always wanted. It's all possible!

Past Life Bullying Affected Deborah's Child

Social anxiety from bullying is a huge problem in modern society. Bullying is a big topic in the news because it seems incredibly unenlightened for modern people to treat each other so poorly. Knowing someone is out to get you by purposefully attempting to instill fear is cause for great stress and turmoil in anyone's life.

All of us have likely suffered at the hands of a bully at some point in our past. Even I had someone who used intimidation tactics on me at every turn. I can't even tell you what caused this person to come after me in the first place because as far as I was concerned, I didn't do anything specific to initiate it, at least *not in this lifetime*. Then again, I had to wonder: Did the bully and I have unresolved karma?

That's a question my client Deborah asked when she came in for a regression and wound up telling me all about one of the other mothers in her child's class at school whose older son teased her little boy non-stop about his thick glasses. The constant torment overshadowed his sweet personality and caused her son to become so withdrawn at school, he stopped socializing with his usual friends. The two moms served together in the elementary school PTA and were at each other's throats all the time. After Deborah repeatedly complained to the principal about the bullying, nothing changed.

"My son can't help the fact that he wears glasses. He doesn't deserve to be treated like this. I have a horrible feeling about *that woman* (his mother). I'm worried because every time I see her I want to punch her and I know if I actually do that, I could get into big trouble, and my son will suffer. As it is, we've been in the principal's office too many times to count, and I'm sick of it. I just need it to stop. I'm a nice person, really I am! I don't normally act like this! I swear I've never had anything like this happen to me before. I told my husband I have a terrible feeling this woman is out to get me. I can't shake it, so I'm here to see if I can get answers before I do something I'll regret, or before her boy does something to my son. If that happens, I know for sure I won't be able to contain myself. I can hardly control myself now. I can't sleep, I've lost my appetite, and every time I have to go to one of those meetings, I freak out. I can't keep going with things the way they are. We could pull my son out of school and take him somewhere else, but I don't believe in that. He shouldn't have to change schools because of an older kid torturing him, and who's to say it wouldn't happen somewhere else? I have to solve this problem here, where we are now."

We visited her past life, and sure enough, these two had a connection— and not a good one.

SK: Go back to the source event where you first knew the soul of this woman. Be there now. What year is this?

Deborah: Somewhere in Europe.

SK: What year is this?

Deborah: 1389. This is weird, but I am a man.

SK: Very good. Are you alone or with other people in 1389 Europe?

Deborah: Right now, I am alone on a road.

SK: Fast forward to a time when you're with other people. Be there now and tell me what's going on.

Deborah: I walked down that road to the center of a village. There's a mob there and someone is being punished.

SK: Is there anyone you know from your current life?

Deborah: Oh yes. She's there. That's her.

SK: What is your relationship in that life?

Deborah: I knew her from the town. Now she's being punished along with her kids for stealing food. They're all taken into the center of town and shackled to some wooden post. Everyone's gathering around, including me. I pick up a stone and throw it, hitting her kid in the head. She looks me right in the eye.

SK: What happens to them?

Deborah: They're all killed. We stoned them. They died a horrible death.

SK: Imagine you can bring them out in front of you now and apologize for doing this to them. Tell them you were only going along with the crowd.

Deborah: That's just it, I hate to admit this, but I enjoyed it. I wasn't a nice person. I didn't have to be there that day. I *wanted* to be there. I wanted to participate. I'm not sure why. I liked the feeling of control back then.

SK: How is that life affecting you in the now?

Deborah: I grew up with all brothers who were hunters and I never liked them hunting. I think it has to do with this life. I don't want to be part of brutality anymore. I've learned over the centuries that fighting and going against others isn't right.

SK: Were there other lifetimes when you fought other people and tortured them?

Deborah: Yes.

SK: Be there now. Notice what's happening.

Deborah: This is also in Europe in the 1700s. This feels more like England, but now that I think about it, the other place was around France. I witnessed a lot of hangings. It was a bad time, lots of poor people, and crime was on the rise.

SK: When you look around at the people in England in the 1700s, do you recognize anyone there from your current life?

Deborah: No.

SK: Were there any events in your past where you received punishment?

Deborah: Yes, long ago.

SK: Be there now. What year is this?

Deborah: I want to say this is in the times of the Romans. I don't have the details, but my guide is showing me I was tortured there. Stabbed and left for dead.

SK: What crime did you commit?

Deborah: Nothing too bad. Stealing food. Same as the people I tortured. You didn't have to do much back in those times when food was scarce to receive death as a punishment.

SK: Did you pay any of those people back who executed you?

Deborah: Oh yes, I think there's been some back and forth with paybacks. I just want to call it even now, though, and be done.

SK: Imagine you can bring the mother of the little boy out in front of you, along with her son and your son in this life. Go ahead and apologize to her for the stoning and see what she says.

Deborah: She doesn't forgive me.

SK: What could you do to change this?

Deborah: She says she's enjoyed watching my son suffer because I watched her child suffer and it feels good.

SK: Were there other lifetimes where you two knew each other?

Deborah: No.

SK: What about your two sons?

Deborah: No. She's saying it's taken a long time to finally get even with me for what I did.

SK: Allow your spirit guide to come in and act as an intermediary between the two of you. Is there any compromise here? Anything you can do to help?

Deborah: My guide says I need to go up to her and apologize. That doesn't make any sense. She's not going to know what I am talking about, but my guide says I have to do this in person in order to heal.

Many times, the person can do the healing in the unified field, in their mind, and real results take hold in the outer world by healing on the inside. In this case, however, for whatever reason, Deborah left feeling clearly guided that she needed to initiate some sort of apology for something she did not do in this lifetime. A week later she told me:

"I couldn't believe what happened after our session. I took a few deep breaths and tried putting myself in her shoes and went up to her after a PTA meeting. I could not get that image of her baby being stoned out of my mind and I whispered into her ear, 'I'm sorry for all you're going through.' She turned around and had the strangest look on her face. I've never seen anything like it. Her eyes welled up and she almost cried. She actually thanked me and apologized. She explained that she and her husband had separated and planned to divorce. She regretted not doing more to stop her son. She tried talking to him, but he was upset about what was happening at home, too, and she had run out of energy to discipline him. Once we talked, everything changed. We're kind of friends now. Well, that might be stretching it a bit, but she goes out of her way to say hi in the carpool lines and my boy hasn't had a single complaint since. I'm thinking of inviting them over after school soon so the two of them can play. I can't even believe I'm saying this, but everything changed and things are looking up."

When you shift your attitude about people, they have to change to conform to your new thinking. Many times bullies wind up being frail underneath their rough exteriors, as Deborah discovered. The bully's perceived anger and rude behavior isn't always personal and is normally a cover-up for troubles in their own lives. When we can show compassion, things change.

Deborah's experience is similar to what I experienced with my bully. I shifted my thinking from fear to tolerance and held my ground against the unwanted behavior. Once I changed, we had a long-overdue conversation and became friends. Know with a little extra compassion and time, things can turn around even in the most difficult situations.

Michelle Constantly Worried About Her Son

Separation anxiety is very real and can become quite problematic. During Michelle's session, she told me she experienced constant nightmares about her third-grade son. She started every day trembling from anxiety before putting him on his school bus. I asked her if something had happened to make her feel this way.

"Not at all," she told me with tears in her eyes. "I just can't shake the feeling that something horrible is going to happen to him, even though we have a nice life, his father is a good man, and there's no logical reason for me to be so upset, but I can't help it."

Was Michelle suffering from feelings carried over from a past life? I wanted to find out.

Sure enough, Michelle recalled a past life in early twentieth-century Chicago. To her surprise and mine, she saw herself as a little girl and her son as her father. The family lived in the city, and one day when the little girl walked to school with her father nearby, a car struck and killed her. It broke her father's heart and he never recovered.

SK: What lessons did you and your son come here to learn about in many lifetimes?

Michelle: He decided to come back again because he wants us to spend a longer time together this lifetime.

SK: Very good. Go ahead and bring out the little girl you were back then, your father from that lifetime, and your son. Imagine this is your son's Higher Self, his soul. Go ahead and speak to them now about these lessons and whether or not you can choose differently this time.

Michelle: Yes, we definitely can. We've agreed to come back to the Chicago area again and this time around we will do better.

SK: Can you see there was no mistake in what happened?

Michelle: Yes.

SK: What lessons did you receive from the accident?

Michelle: There wasn't really a lesson. I had to go early, up to … heaven, I guess you'd call it. I had some spiritual training to do.

SK: Is that training helping you in your current life?

Michelle: (laughing) I hope it can now, but so far, not so much. I need to stop my worry and let go of fear. This is all an illusion. We are infinite, so there is nothing to worry about.

SK: Very good. So do you think you can have a successful and lengthy life together this time around?

Michelle: Oh yes, we will. But I have to stop the worrying or my son won't want to be around me and he won't be properly prepared to face the world. He needs to be strong, and he can't be unless I become stronger.

SK: Are you ready to do that?

Michelle: Yes, definitely.

Once the two parties solidified the agreement, Michelle traveled to her current-life future and saw the family years later.

SK: Where are you now?

Michelle: My son's graduation from college.

SK: How do you feel?

Michelle: Great. Everything worked out this time around and we still have a wonderful relationship.

SK: As you experience yourself in the future, imagine you can look back over your life and notice when you let go of your anxiety about your son.

Michelle: I did that today.

SK: Nice. Are you able and willing to let go of your anxiety about his safety? At least for the most part?

Michelle: I can.

SK: When will you do that?

Michelle: Now.

She spoke with conviction, so we had only one more step to do.

SK: Great. Now go back to your son's graduation and really tune in to the feeling you have now that he has safely graduated. Allow every cell in your body to relax knowing he is fine and he is safe. Allow your subconscious mind to give you a symbol that represents your new feeling of calm where your son is concerned. What is that symbol?

Michelle: A graduation cap.

Once she identified the graduation cap as her symbol for her newfound peace, she used the hat to trigger reassured thoughts for her future.

In part three of this book, you'll get to discover a powerful healing symbol of your own. For Michelle, from that day on, she became empowered to create the life she wanted to live, rather than being stuck in a painful pattern of misery.

SK: Every time you think about a graduation cap or you see one on television or in a movie, anywhere at all, you will instantly be brought back into the memory of your son's graduation and you will know that all is well and he is doing great. Any other insights or lessons you received?

Michelle: We are not stuck here on Earth. There's more that we can't see. We are going on from here. There is no death of our spirit, so we are okay, no matter what.

Sometimes a little understanding goes a long way. Many times, our unexplained emotions aren't actually caused by anything we are or are not doing in our current lives, and yet this is often hard to determine because we are so invested in the illusion of three-dimensional consciousness. In Michelle's case, she was truly surprised to realize roles were reversed in the past, but by simply observing that, accepting what happened in the last life she and her son shared, she easily let go of her anxiety. Last I heard from her, she had never looked back.

Panic

Panic attacks, according to DSM-5, have several symptoms and must be "associated with longer than one month of subsequent persistent worry about having another attack or consequences of the attack."

Earlier in the book I mentioned a fascinating phenomenon I call *Supretrovie*, or spontaneous past life memories brought on by external stimuli. I've discovered thousands of people have memories of prior incarnations that are triggered by external events—places they visit, people they see, or physical objects. These memories often trigger traumatic reactions in the present. When people experience *Supretrovie*, they often require a past life regression, not to identify the prior lifetime, but to go back into the situation in a safe environment so they can heal the trauma and get on with their lives. Many people have past life memories spontaneously pop up while they are traveling. These situations are different from déjà vu because they are not examples of knowing you've had the same exact experience repeated, but instead, you remember a long-forgotten time on a conscious level, of something you did in the past, or of the place you're visiting. These experiences often cause tremendous panic and anxiety, yet when the events are happening, people are not always aware that the trauma is being caused by a past life in that area.

Kyle Feared the Nile

Kyle believed he had definitely lived a past life in Egypt after he went to Cairo on business and became incredibly fearful.

"We were in the city center and I was with my colleagues walking along the sidewalk next to the Nile, not too far from the Egyptian National Museum. We were about to cross over the river when we decided to stop and glance down at the Nile. For some reason, a profound sense of terror overwhelmed me. I almost started to cry when I saw the water. It wasn't a sad cry; it was angrier, like something wicked had happened there. Something I hadn't thought about for a very long time. I held my breath and tried to get myself under control because I didn't want my coworkers to see me. I wanted to run, but I froze from fear and couldn't move for a second. I tried breathing and after a few minutes, by the time my coworkers approached, I could move my legs again. I just stayed quiet while we walked back to the hotel and averted my eyes so I wouldn't have to see the Nile. I stared at the sidewalk until I could get myself under control. Once I got back to the hotel lobby, they all wanted to go eat, but I said no and went to my room. Seeing that place wore me out. I showered and went to bed, but that terrible feeling from the Nile lingered. I didn't cry; I rarely do. I've never experienced such bad vibes before or since. I'll never forget that as long as I live."

I could certainly understand feeling emotional after visiting a place. I've even felt that way after meeting certain people I believe I've known in past lives. You may have had similar experiences. Nevertheless, I was excited to learn about Kyle's connection to Egypt, so we did the regression.

SK: Where are you and what year is it?

Kyle: I'm in Egypt sometime before the pyramids were built. I don't know the date.

SK: What's happening?

Kyle: I am with hundreds of people. We are doing some kind of ritual along the Nile. There is fire, smoke, a ceremony.

SK: Are you a man or a woman?

Kyle: Man.

SK: As you experience the energy of the people there, what is your relationship to them?

Kyle: I sense a woman there. I love her. We are together, although not formally. I know there is some ritual that must be performed. Not too different from marriage, but it's more religious than that. I promised we will be together.

SK: Is she there with you at this ceremony?

Kyle: Yes.

SK: Surrounded by healing light, go to the event that is the source event for the strange feeling you had when you were in Cairo. Be there now, notice what's happening.

Kyle: She's performing a risky ritual along the banks of the river. I don't like it, but it is commanded by the rulers at the time that she obey. She missteps and slips and falls, hitting her head. I'm watching as her body floats down the river. People are holding me back. I want to dive in and get her, but they say no, I cannot. I am needed elsewhere. I fought and was restrained and sent away, brokenhearted and angry. I became convinced the Pharaoh was evil after that and his ways were not pure. I was eventually put to death for my disobedience.

SK: How is this life affecting you now?

Kyle: It wasn't until I traveled back there that I realized I do have a tendency to be a rebel at work. I've missed a lot of opportunities because I refuse to do what I'm told. I stress myself out over things when I don't feel they're fair.

SK: Imagine you can be back on the Nile and notice a loving, healing light coming down from above, washing away your sorrow and bitterness. Allow that light to move into your heart, releasing you from this energy so you are more open to receive. Let me know when this feels better.

> *Kyle:* Yes, although part of my soul will still never get over what they did to her. I could have easily saved her if they would have just let me go help. I have a hard time with that still.

I've found past life regression to be incredibly helpful for coming to a state of acceptance about some of the injustices in the world. Forgiveness and letting go are hard for each of us for different reasons. Kyle's story is a great example of something I describe as peeling back the layers of the onion of your subconscious mind, only to realize there's much more to go in the future. Some things we will never accept, no matter what, but having the clarity can still provide some degree of healing.

New Orleans Haunted House Panicked Erin

One of the more interesting regressions I've done involved Erin, who couldn't shake the spooky vibes she picked up from a haunted house. Here's what happened:

"I live in Los Angeles and I went to New Orleans over Halloween one year to meet some girlfriends who live on the East Coast. We went on one of those ghost tours of the Garden District, and I got really spooked in one of the houses. I didn't see anything, like I didn't see a ghost or spirit, but I felt terrorized there, to the point I could hardly sleep that night. My friends thought it was funny, which I don't blame them for, but if they could have been inside my head, they would have known this fear was real. Down-to-the-bone real. Bad enough I didn't get any sleep and had nightmares all night. The following day when we went back to that area for a tour, I started hyperventilating in the downstairs lobby of one of those mansions. My heart raced so fast I thought it was going to pop out of my chest. Thank God, I managed to make it to a sofa and sit down before I fell down. It was really bad. I was sweating and I couldn't catch my breath. I thought I was going to die. I felt super embarrassed when one of my friends came over and tried to get me to calm down, which I did to some degree. I missed out on Bourbon Street and partying that night, because my friends were worried there might really be something wrong with me, like I think they thought I had the flu. I went to my hotel room and went straight to bed and felt fine. The next day I flew home, no problem, but I've always believed I picked up some bad juju from that haunted place—a spirit or something that stuck with me—because ever since then, when I think about New Orleans, I get a bad vibe."

During her past life regression, Erin definitely uncovered a connection to the New Orleans area.

SK: What year is it, the first thing that comes to your mind?

Erin: 1700s, but I don't know the exact date.

SK: Where are you and what's happening?

Erin: I'm in a mansion.

SK: Visiting or do you live there?

Erin: I live there in that same area where we went, only there's nothing else around.

The key to Erin's challenges happened at the end of her prior incarnation.

SK: Fast forward to the very last day of your life and tell me how it is you pass into spirit.

Erin: I'm very old. I'm fixing food when my heart starts racing and I fall down in the kitchen. I'm having a heart attack. I die.

SK: Go ahead and lift up, up, up, out of that body, out of that life. Surrounded by a healing light, notice if these symptoms you experienced in the mansion lobby are similar to what you experienced in the 1700s.

Erin: They're just the same, only I wasn't going to die.

SK: Very good. Imagine you can speak to the Higher Self of the woman you were back then. Notice there's an energetic cord connecting the two of you and in a moment, when I count down from three, we're going to cut that cord, releasing and healing you from those events in your past. Ready? Three, two, one, cut! Notice there's now a healing light pouring into your heart, relaxing and healing you. Let me know when this feels better.

Erin: It's definitely better now.

Before her regression, Erin mentioned her concerns regarding the possibility that she inadvertently picked up some wandering souls from the mansions she had visited. I refer to them as *stragglers*, and they could have definitely caused her to feel fearful. I've worked with dozens of people negatively affected by discarnate beings over the years, so I asked her about that:

> *SK:* Did any of the spirits in New Orleans come home with you?
>
> *Erin:* No. That's what I thought originally, but now I realize I was just sensitive to the energy because I had lived there before.

Incredibly, we can energetically carry over medical issues and conditions from the past into our current lives, especially in cases like Erin's, where she had actually visited a place where she'd been long ago. With a few simple shifts, Erin changed everything.

Summing Up

All of the case studies explored in this chapter show how debilitating panic and anxiety can be in normal waking life. When challenges won't quit, that's when it's time to look into the past for answers.

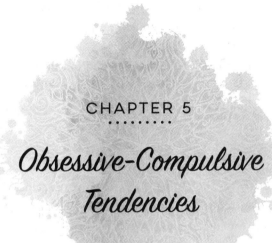

CHAPTER 5
· · · · · · · · ·

Obsessive-Compulsive Tendencies

LET'S BE HONEST WITH ourselves, shall we? Everybody is weird. We all have idiosyncrasies that other people would find more than a little bit strange. So while we aren't here to self-diagnose or judge, this next section will delve into some of the bizarre behavior I've witnessed with clients over the years. Who knows? Maybe you'll see a little bit of yourself in some of these individuals. I know I have. We're all one, after all ...

Obsessive Compulsive Disorder

DSM-5 states Obsessive Compulsive Disorder involves a "presence of obsessions, compulsions, or both."

Obsessions involve recurrent, persistent thoughts and urges, while compulsions are repetitive behaviors. We all have some of these tendencies, but when they go to extremes and nothing else helps, perhaps it's time to look into a past life experience for answers.

Claudia Became a Cat Lady Thanks to Her Past Life Promise

Thanks to the hit A&E television show *Hoarders*, this phenomenon is now widely known by the general public. The effects can be devastating on both finances and health. According to the DSM-5, hoarders are officially defined as "individuals who excessively save items and [to whom] the idea of discarding items causes extreme stress."

Like many of the strange behaviors discussed in this book, hoarding could have root causes either in past lives or in the client's current life. Typically, when we think of hoarding, people imagine piles of useless junk stuffed into every nook and cranny, but one of my more memorable cases involved a completely different kind of hoarding.

Claudia served on the Board of Directors for her local animal shelter and volunteered regularly for the Humane Society. She constantly fought for animal rights by raising funds and awareness in an area of the country known for vocal advocates for such matters. By all accounts, Claudia was a pillar of her community and a credit to humanity, a friend to many, and a gift to all who knew her, especially the four-legged friends she assisted throughout her incredible journey.

When we met at one of my seminars and Claudia wanted to do a private session, I couldn't imagine it would be about anything more than curiosity, because the woman seemed to have it all together. She easily traveled back in time to her past life in an Egyptian cult. Unlike the modern connotation, in ancient times, dedicated worshipers tended a deity of their choosing by making daily offerings and performing rituals. In Claudia's case, her cult had direct connections with her current passion for animals.

SK: Where are you and what's happening?

Claudia: We're in a special group who worship the goddess Bastet, the cat.

SK: Very good. What kinds of rituals do you observe there?

Claudia: We must care for the cats, feeding them, tending to them to ensure no harm ever comes to them.

Cats were sacred to all ancient Egyptians, but particularly so to members of the Bastet cult. My client went into a vision where she saw her duty in great detail, including the promise she had made long ago.

Claudia: I am a priestess.

SK: What lessons did you learn as an Egyptian priestess, and how do those lessons apply to your life now?

I ask that question a lot, and I expected her to mention her work at the Humane Society and other wonderful deeds she'd done. Instead, she shocked me by bursting into tears and coming completely out of her hypnotic state.

SK: What's wrong?

Claudia: I have to tell you something. I'm not what everybody thinks I am.

She explained that she had moved to her current home five years earlier after being accused of animal hoarding. The accusation and punishment ruined her reputation as a rescue agency.

Claudia: It was awful. I didn't mean to do it, but at one point, I'd taken in over a hundred cats and the conditions in my house were … unmanageable, to say the least.

She explained that a court reassigned her cats to other caregivers and she had paid hefty fines.

Claudia: It's been really hard. (still crying) Even though I know I can't have them, I have a constant thought in my mind about taking one, or two, or three, and keeping them for myself, caring for the cats the way I know they deserve. The problem is that once I start inviting them in, I can't stop, so I try to control the urge.

You can see how Claudia's past life love for cats caused controversy in her current life. Later in the book, I'll share what else I uncovered when we went deeper into her Egyptian incarnation and how we finally got to the bottom of the situation. For now, let's take a look at some more interesting but strange cases.

David Couldn't Sit Because His Life Depended on It

I've been blessed to find a number of interesting cases over the years. Certainly one of the most memorable involved David, who came to see me after being fired from his job at a bank.

David had found new employment at a warehouse distribution center and said the work suited him better because he had an opportunity to move around more in that job. I concurred that sitting behind a desk can be tiring, and that's when the real issue emerged.

"Actually, that's why I was fired," David explained. "I wouldn't sit at my desk."

"Were you afraid to sit?" I asked.

"No. It felt more like a force compelling me so I could not sit no matter how hard I tried. If I sat for a moment, to rest, then I knew I had to hurry so I would stand up as soon as I could."

"Is this still happening?"

"Oh yes. That's why I'm here, among other reasons."

"But you did not feel driven by fear?"

"No. I couldn't stand being stuck at a desk all day. I'm claustrophobic."

We talked about his early life and I wondered if he had been trapped inside an enclosed space or had been a victim of some other accident of some kind. Apparently, he had an obsession with standing. I say *obsession* because we all might like to get up to stretch our legs once in a while, but according to his accounts, he couldn't sit, not even for a moment, which made things quite difficult when he worked with clients who came into the bank to see him about loans. I wondered how David could have possibly made it through college and he explained that he attended an online university and that this was his first real job out of school.

"They wrote me up, then fired me," he explained.

"Do you have a medical condition that explains this? Maybe you can receive restitution."

"No. I've been to doctors. There's nothing wrong with me. That's why I'm here."

I hear that a lot from people—they come in to see me as a last resort when nothing makes sense and they've tried everything else.

Fortunately, David was open to past lives. I wanted to at least attempt to take him there, and to his childhood. I thought perhaps he had been punished or ridiculed for sitting at some tender age. When I asked him to return to the source event of his difficulty, David went back to a horrific moment in World War II.

SK: What year is this? The first thing that comes to your mind.

David: 1938.

SK: And where are you in the world?

David: Germany.

SK: What's happening?

David: I'm in a building crowded with people. They're shouting and everyone is shoving and pushing. The smell is horrible.

SK: Why are they shoving?

David: They don't mean to. We have to hurry.

His voice trailed off and he became silent for a minute.

SK: What's happening now?

David: People are still shoving. We're going outside. It's cold. We have to work.

SK: What are you working on?

David: Don't know. We're carrying heavy poles across a field. Some are falling down.

He gasped.

SK: What happened?

David: Someone started to fall. They shot him, and then they shot another person for no reason.

Silent for quite a while, David began trembling. A tear trickled down his cheek.

David: I see them.

SK: Who?

David: Officers. They're shoving us. We're so tired. And hungry. It's hard to work. (gasping again) Another one fell. She was too weak to walk. They put a bullet in her head.

After establishing a protected space, David floated above the events and moved toward the very last day of this terrible life.

SK: Surrounded by a protective light, knowing you are safe and secure, notice how it is that you pass into spirit.

David: I am walking, and I trip and fall. I look up at the soldier, begging him, but he shoots me anyway. (gasps) Oh my God! He was my boss at my last job!

SK: Go ahead now and float up, out of that body, out of that life. You are safe now in that peaceful space in between lives. What lessons did you learn in Germany?

David: Sometimes you do your best, but things are out of your control.

SK: How is that affecting your current life?

David: I can't sit. I'm afraid to sit. Ever since I went to work at that bank and saw him again, he's messed me up.

SK: So, you're saying you used to be able to sit until you met your boss?

David: I never liked sitting. I can't ever be pinned down, but it got so much worse when I went to work there.

SK: Very good. Now imagine you can invite the person you were then to come and speak to who you are now. Notice there is an energetic cord connecting the two of you. Go ahead and talk to the young man in 1938. Imagine he can talk to you about the fact that you are safe now and it's okay to sit down. Nothing will happen. Then imagine the soldier and your former boss could come up to you. Imagine the soldier could apologize to you.

David: He says he was following orders.

SK: Very good. So, imagine your boss's Higher Self talking to your Higher Self, and he is apologizing.

David: He doesn't need to. He didn't do anything wrong to me this time. I messed up. I am sorry.

SK: Very good. Notice if there are other lifetimes when the two of you knew each other. Yes or no?

David: Oh yes.

SK: Go ahead and float over those events in the 1930s and imagine you can turn back toward the past. In a moment, when I count to three, you will arrive at the source event or the most important event that is affecting the two of you. One, two, three. Be there now. Where are you?

David's whole demeanor changed. He visibly strengthened.

David: I'm a soldier.

SK: What year is this? The first thing that comes to your mind.

David: (after a moment) Not sure ...

SK: What part of the world are you in?

David: I am a Roman, a Roman soldier.

SK: Good job. Imagine you can move through your life as a soldier until you reach the most important event that shows you your connection to your former boss. Be there now and tell me what's happening.

David: We are plundering a village. Killing everyone we see.

SK: And is your former boss there?

David: Yes. He's a little boy. I shot him.

SK: Why did you do it?

David: I had to. If I didn't, I would have been shot myself. (After a moment of silence.) I get it now. He did to me what I did to him earlier. He had to kill me in Germany or he would have died, and even in this life, his boss made him fire me. I talked to him a lot and he tried to give

me a chance, but after I wouldn't change, he had no choice but to let
me go.

SK: Very good. Do you think you can let this go now?

David: Yes.

SK: When do you want to let this go?

David: Now.

SK: Very good. Bring the Roman soldier and the little boy out and have
them meet with the Nazi and the boy you were then, and bring out
your former boss. Notice there are energetic cords connecting all of
you. In a moment when I count down from three, an angel will cut
those cords and release all of you in a spirit of forgiveness. You were all
doing the best you could at the time. Ready? Three, two, one, cut the
cords!

David cut the cords and I did some energy healing on him until he reported
feeling lighter and better. During his regression, David experienced a true epiphany and seemed to accept the healing. Still, the only way to know for sure if
hypnotic intervention is successful is by observing how the person gets along in
the real world.

Clearly David realized he no longer needed to hang on to old fears about
sitting down. In daily life, he would hopefully notice the change the moment
he took a seat at work.

David's situation is a great example of why it is imperative to have the
client travel out to their current life future to experience themselves happily
free from their worries. In this case, David visited a future event that reconfirmed he had made the change:

David: I'm at work and I'm eating lunch with my coworkers.

SK: Where do you work?

David: The same place I do now. I still enjoy it.

SK: Are you standing or sitting?

David: Sitting with my friends at one of the benches outside behind the
building.

SK: How do you feel?

David: It's a sunny day and I feel great.

We did another exercise to get David fully engaged in the feeling of relaxation while seated.

I don't always hear from past clients, but in this case, I asked David to keep in touch. A little over a year later, he contacted me to say:

"I'm better than ever and I never had a problem sitting ever again."

It's a good feeling to know this helped. Change is real, it is possible, and it all begins in the mind.

Antonio's Itchy Skin Began in a Past Life

Antonio suffered from kidney failure and during the last years of his life, he began picking his skin. Itching is common for people in his situation, so everyone assumed the habit was caused by his illness or an allergic reaction to one of the many drugs he took. After several energy healing and regression sessions, we accidentally discovered more to Antonio's itching than we had thought:

SK: Where are you and what year is this?

Antonio: I'm in Europe. Middle Ages or some very dark time. The stench is unbelievable, the living conditions are horrible. I'm basically a bum and I beg for food and ale from the local watering hole. There's an infestation of bugs going around. They're biting everybody, absolutely miserable. Nobody bathes, though, and it seems like this is normal.

SK: Imagine you can float up and out of that body in the Middle Ages and notice an energetic cord connecting you with the person you were back then. In a moment, we will cut that cord and free you from that energy. Three, two, one, cutting that cord. A healing light is bathing your skin, removing the bugs. Imagine they are evaporating into thin air. Take your time and let me know when they're completely gone.

Antonio: (after a minute) Yes, they're gone now.

SK: Good job. Notice a beautiful healing light relieving your itching, healing any irritated parts of your skin, and bringing peace. Let me know when this feels better to you.

Antonio: (after a minute) Yes. I am better.

I did some research into Antonio's story and the Middle Ages were, in fact, notorious for lice, which were actually considered lucky at the time. Incredibly, people observed that sick people rarely had lice, so if you had them, you were less likely to contract the plague, and therefore considered fortunate. The process did not completely remedy Antonio's itching, but it did help somewhat, since his itching really was partially caused by his medications. Still, knowing he felt a bit better than before the session was a huge victory.

Cynthia Had a Perfect Nose in Her Prior Life

There probably isn't a person alive who is one hundred percent happy with every single thing about their body or the way they look. We all have a few hang-ups here and there, and that's natural . . . until it isn't.

One rare Obsessive Compulsive Disorder is called Body Dysmorphic Disorder, defined by the DSM-5 as "distress due to a perceived physical anomaly, such as a scar, the shape or size of a body part, or some other personal feature."

In her mid-forties, Cynthia came to see me for a regression and discovered a deep truth about herself while receiving an unexpected healing. When I work with my clients, I use my intuition to sense where they need to go in terms of guided imagery. There are hundreds of different variations of a regression that I can take people on, and for Cynthia, I was clearly guided to use a more traditional and typical method—a long walk down the stairs and into a closet. As you can imagine, I don't always use this imagery because many people are afraid of enclosed spaces and closets in general. In this case, that method was exactly what Cynthia needed.

Once Cynthia reached the closet, she stepped inside and tried on some clothes, glanced in a mirror, and immediately burst into tears.

SK: What's wrong? Where are you?

Cynthia: (crying) It's perfect!

SK: Tell me what you mean.

Cynthia: My nose. (Brings her hands up to her face and touches her nose.) It's beautiful.

Still not fully comprehending the magnitude of what she was going through, I prompted further.

SK: Go ahead and continue looking at your beautiful nose in the mirror and, as you do, you will see there is a doorknob on that mirror. Turn the knob, open the door, and walk out into your life with your beautiful nose. Be there now and notice what's happening. What year is it, the first thing that comes to your mind?

Cynthia: 1729.

SK: Very good. And where are you in the world?

Cynthia: France.

SK: What are you doing in France in 1729?

Cynthia: I am in the French court, very wealthy and beautiful.

She reported being married to a wealthy landowner and courtier of King Louis XV. I asked if there were people there who were with her in her current life, and she said no, but she found one important connection.

Cynthia: My looks were so perfect then. I've tried to get back to that in my current life, but I haven't been successful. I wanted to have my nose fixed ever since I was ten.

Once she returned to waking consciousness, she seemed to be at greater internal peace about herself and accepted her current-life appearance as not only adequate but, as she said herself, *"beautiful in my own way."*

When there is something on the outside that is not pleasing us, it might be better to look on the inside for answers. Unless the inside changes, there is no amount of outer work that can be done to improve someone.

Using guided imagery and positive affirmations is key to success in many areas of life, and for Cynthia, a trip into her past proved hugely beneficial. I ran into her again some time later and although we were in a public venue and did not have a chance to speak privately, she seemed more at ease with herself than when we first met.

Jeff's Girlfriend Scared Him to Death

Another possible manifestation of OCD is Obsessive Love Disorder. Although it's not officially recognized in the DSM-5 as a named condition, according to Healthline.com, Obsessive Love Disorder is a very real issue involving unhealthy attachments to others.[5]

I've been fascinated over the years by a concept I call *Karmic Obsession*, which is the idea that we definitely meet our karma when we're inexplicably drawn in unhealthy ways to individuals from our deep past. I suspected karmic obsession was to blame for Jeff's problems when he told me he had a deep fear whenever he was around his girlfriend.

"Is she abusive?" I asked.

"No, not at all. I just don't feel right around her."

We discussed the fact that he should probably leave her or end the relationship if it caused him to feel so uneasy.

He insisted that wasn't an option. "I can't stop seeing her. I know that doesn't make any sense, but I can't leave her. From the moment I laid eyes on her, I had to be with her. She wanted nothing to do with me when we first met and I had to work hard to get her to date me, so now that I have her, even though she doesn't always treat me the way I want and rejected me more times than I want to admit, I can't let go of her now. I keep hoping things will get better."

> *SK:* Go to the source event where you and your girlfriend first met. Where are you?
>
> *Jeff:* England, 1600s. I'm a knight and she is my love. I die defending her honor even though she rejected me. I thought I could win her over by fighting, but it didn't work out.

• • • • • • • • • • • • •

5. Cherney, Kristeen and Timothy J. Legg, PhD, "Obsessive Love Disorder: What is Obsessive Love Disorder?" Healthline.com, January 10, 2018. https://www.healthline.com /health/obsessive-love-disorder

In order for the RELIEF Method to work, the client must return to the very first event in time. Intuitively, I felt Jeff hadn't gone back that far yet, so I asked him again, and sure enough, he confirmed he had not accessed the earliest lifetime he and his girlfriend had shared.

SK: Was your life in England the source event of your challenges?

Jeff: No.

SK: I want you to go back in time to the first time, the source event, where the two of you first met and be there now and tell me what you see.

Jeff: I'm a cave man.

SK: Very good. When is this?

Jeff: Early, before recorded history.

SK: And what is the connection between you and your girlfriend when you were a caveman?

Jeff: She's my mate again and I'm trying to save her from some animal, but I get killed and she runs off to safety, into the arms of another man in our tribe.

SK: Very good. How do these lives relate to the things you're doing together in your current life?

Jeff: She's very chaotic, even now. I do all I can to try to save her by helping her with things, but in the end, I lose. She doesn't always act like she's interested in me at all, like there's something better waiting for her around the corner. Even in those other lives, she had other people she wanted more than me, and I tried to prove I was worth it, only she didn't care. The same thing's happening now. I may not die, but if I stay with her, I'll wind up with nothing but disappointment.

After doing some energy healing around the situation, in the end, Jeff reconfirmed what he already knew—he needed to end the unhealthy relationship. It seemed obvious this supposed girlfriend did not see Jeff in the same light as he viewed her, and things hadn't changed much between them over the thousands of years they'd known each other. Jeff understood he had free will to either expunge himself from the toxic relationship by basically following his own advice and discontinuing contact with her or stay and take his chances on another heartache.

Karmic Obsessions are incredibly common in my private practice. Clients often ask me what I think. "Should I stay with him/her?" My answer is always the same—if you have to ask, unfortunately, you probably already know the answer. We all have the innate wisdom and common sense within our souls to know what we should do in any given situation, and my heart goes out to people who are struggling with these issues. We've all been there with someone in our lives. These conflicts are yet another way we meet our own karma coming and going.

As for Jeff, I'm not sure what happened, but I certainly hope he found peace. In the end, it's all about choice and every single one of us has the free will to choose our experiences in this life and all our other lives.

Summing Up

We all have our own eccentricities and often those are intricately linked to the past. It's not always easy to see ourselves enough to know when our behavior is unbalanced, so I applaud my clients for the level of self-analysis they endured to get to the bottom of some incredibly challenging issues.

CHAPTER 6
· · · · · · · · ·
Trauma & Post-Traumatic Stress

THE FOLLOWING SECTION WILL include case studies of people struggling with trauma and post-traumatic stress, which we've unfortunately seen a lot of these days. Between all the extreme weather events, and unbelievable struggles our men and women in uniform have endured after returning from horrific scenes on the battlefield, people are stressed beyond belief for a wide variety of reasons. Although I've never been involved in the military or warzones in my current life, my heart goes out to our service members as well as all those who suffer extreme trauma. Once you witness certain things, they can be quite difficult, if not impossible, to forget.

One of most common traumatic situations I deal with in my practice is helping those who suffer from grief. All human beings will suffer some kind of loss in their lives. While the pain of grief is staggering, you can learn to gain greater acceptance about loss and other distressing events. Hypnotherapy, and past life regression in particular, can be a true blessing and a relief for those who suffer from a trauma or post-traumatic stress by helping people view tragedies in new ways.

Trauma

Trauma is a very complex diagnosis involving several key factors. According to the DSM-5, trauma is defined as "exposure to actual or threatened death, serious injury, or sexual violence."

Thankfully none of the next case histories will involve anything so dire, but when lingering feelings of death carry over in soul memory from centuries ago, the result can often feel devastating unless a major paradigm shift occurs.

Pam Couldn't Commit

Adopted children who grow up in unstable environments and bounce from one foster home to another often understandably develop post-traumatic stress. Like any taxing situation, painful emotions can remain buried for years. Pam pushed her memories out of her mind. She got by in life, and did well, but at times, issues reared up in unexpected ways any time Pam began to pursue a relationship.

An incredibly kind girl in her early twenties, Pam seemed the pillar of normalcy. She had a good job that she enjoyed, a nice place to live, and according to her, a wonderful boyfriend who wanted to become her fiancé sooner rather than later. Pam only had one problem—she couldn't bring herself to commit.

Her inability to give her boyfriend an answer when he repeatedly asked Pam to marry him wore the bonds of their relationship dangerously thin, so she decided to see me about emotional healing. Pam expressed extreme and sincere gratitude for her wonderful life. The child of a drug addict, she only spent a very short time in foster care as a baby before getting adopted by her family before the age of three months.

"I am so lucky in my life to have such a loving adoptive family," Pam said. "They always let me know I was adopted and made sure I knew I was loved. I've never wanted for anything. I wasn't raised in harsh conditions at all, but when I think about settling down with Brian, my heart races and I get a sick feeling in my stomach. Fear comes out of nowhere, paralyzing me and making it hard to breathe. I've tried telling Brian this has nothing to do with him, but he says I'm rejecting him, which I'm not. I feel bad. I'm sure this hasn't been good for his ego, and I'm afraid if I can't say yes, he's going to leave me, and then what would I do?"

Thanks to Pam's grateful and receiving attitude, I had faith that with a little help she could have the life she truly wanted. Even if you cannot remember every little detail of your earliest days on Earth, your soul knows exactly what happened. For that reason, we began her session by having her go into the deep past to her birth.

SK: When you think of your birth, what emotion comes to mind?

Pam: Fear.

SK: Very good. Whose fear is this?

Pam: My birth mother. She is afraid of the pain, and now that I'm here, she's afraid of giving me up.

SK: How does that make you feel?

Pam: Well, I never thought much about why she gave me up or what she must have been thinking, so I suppose it is nice to know that on some level, she did care about me.

SK: Very good. Imagine a bright, healing light coming down from above, dissolving your fear. Take your time and let me know when you feel better.

Pam: (After a few minutes.) It's better.

SK: Fast forward in time to your temporary home where you stayed before you were adopted. Be there now and notice what's happening.

Pam: There are a few other children there. I'm the youngest.

SK: How do you feel in that home?

Pam: It's chaos. The other kids all want things; there are toys scattered everywhere.

SK: Are you afraid?

Pam: No. Not at all. There is a sense of caring here. Not love but caring.

SK: Notice a white healing light is covering everyone in the house. Let me know when things feel more peaceful.

Pam: (After a few minutes.) Better.

SK: Fast forward to the moment you were adopted by your new family. Be there now and notice how you feel.

Pam: (emotional, crying) There's so much love. My mom's crying. She's always wanted to have a child and she loves me. She's so happy. My dad too. He's not so emotional normally, but he's choked up.

I thought I would uncover more trauma at her birth or adoption that might translate into her current difficulties with her boyfriend, but things really were fairly good for her compared to other kids in that same situation.

SK: Go back to the source event of your difficulties committing to your boyfriend and be there now.

Pam: I'm in a meadow.

SK: Very good. What year is this?

Pam: 1659?

SK: What part of the world are you in?

Pam: Ireland.

SK: Are you alone or with other people?

Pam: Alone, but I can see my house up ahead.

SK: Go ahead and fast forward to the next time you are in your house with other people and be there now. Notice what's happening. How old are you? Who are you with?

Pam: I'm a young woman, about the same age as I am right now. I am in my house with my infant son and my husband. (crying)

SK: What's wrong?

Pam: My husband's sick. I'm taking care of him. I went to the well to get fresh water to cool his fever, but ... he doesn't make it.

SK: Fast forward to the next most significant event and be there now. Notice what happens next.

Pam: My baby gets sick and dies two days later. I'm sick too. I go to bed, but there's nobody around to take care of me.

SK: Fast forward to the last day of your life in Ireland in the 1600s. Notice how you pass into spirit.

Pam: I don't last much longer. I'm tired and I don't care. I want to die and be with my family.

SK: Go ahead and do that now. Float up into that peaceful space in between lives. Imagine a healing light is moving down over those painful events, washing away your sadness, and let me know when this feels better.

Pam: Yes. It's better.

SK: As you think of your family in Ireland, is there anyone you know in your current lifetime?

Pam: Yes! It's Brian! He was my husband in that life!

SK: How does your life in Ireland relate to your current situation?

Pam: I'm afraid to commit because I can't have my heart broken again. I don't want us to be together only to have him leave me.

SK: Imagine that the man you were married to in Ireland and your boyfriend can come out and stand in front of you. Go ahead and have a conversation with them. What lessons are you here to learn about during these two lifetimes?

Pam: To love unconditionally.

SK: Would it be okay for you to get married in this life, despite what happened in Ireland?

Pam: Yes.

SK: Fast forward to the future in your current life to a moment where you are happy, healthy, and you have successfully experienced your purpose of loving unconditionally and be there now.

Pam: I'm married and we're in our new house. Everything's going well. I'm expecting a baby and our families are happy.

At the end of our session, Pam and I discussed how surprised we both were to find that her difficulty originated in a past life. "I should've known all along it would be okay to marry Brian. I've loved him since the moment we first met."

"No," I said. "You've actually loved him a lot longer than that."

She agreed. Pam's story is a great example of how surprising our past lives can be and why sometimes unexpected sources come up that we would have never realized without taking the journey into other time periods. I received an email from her after she got married and she reported that she and Brian were happy and enjoying their new life together.

Haley Cried on a Cruise Ship

Some people are inexplicably drawn to the ocean, and others, well, let's say they don't like the high seas at all. Perhaps you've heard the Shakespearean quote from *Hamlet* that says: "The lady doth protest too much, methinks."[6] In terms of past life regression or any kind of healing, this phrase exemplifies the simple fact that if you love something a little too much, there might be a past life connection, and likewise, if you absolutely hate something, there's an even better chance of a past life connection. The fine line between love and hate is undoubtedly alive and well in regression therapy, so when someone hates the ocean, I am instantly intrigued. Still, my heart went out to Haley when I heard about her terrible vacation.

"My husband took me on a cruise to the Caribbean for our anniversary. He even bought a suite and everything. He went all-out to make it special, but that first day after we went out to sea, I balled up on my bed in our cabin and cried myself to sleep," she explained. "The ocean was calm, so there wasn't any actual reason for me to act that way, but I was scared to death. My husband felt terrible, like he had caused it, and I felt so bad knowing I'd hurt his feelings, that made me cry even more. Now he's convinced I made the whole thing up. He found a good deal to go to Greece next summer, but the moment he mentioned it, my hands started shaking and I started perspiring. Ever since he mentioned the trip, I've tossed and turned at night, dreading the idea of another cruise. I can't remember any dreams, per se, other than the fact that I don't want to go. What makes me even more anxious is the fact that I didn't have the heart to tell him no, so he's still looking around at prices. Unless I tell him to stop, I'll have to go on this cruise, even though just

. . . .

6. *Hamlet* Quotes, Goodreads.com. https://www.goodreads.com/work/quotes/1885548
   -the-tragicall-historie-of-hamlet-prince-of-denmark.

thinking about it makes me nauseous. I have a bad feeling if I go, I'll die. Isn't that ridiculous? The fear feels worse now than it did on our anniversary, even though we went a few years ago. I have to find answers!"

Haley traveled back in time easily because she meditated regularly and worked on herself over the years. Still, I think she was surprised by what she found in her deep past.

SK: What year is this and where are you?

Haley: Oh … this is strange. It's 1790 and I'm in Europe.

SK: Are you a man or woman?

Before I finished asking her questions, Haley began to cry.

SK: What's happening?

Haley: (crying) This isn't fair, but I'm being put on a ship and taken away for stealing food.

SK: Imagine a bright white light washes over you, protecting you during this journey. Let me know when you feel a little better.

Haley: (crying slows but still sniffling) Yes, I'm better, thanks.

SK: Surrounded by a loving and healing light, knowing that within this light you are safe and secure, imagine you can notice where you are going.

Haley: I don't know. I'm not educated. I'm hungry, so I stole a little bit of something that we would never even think of putting in our mouths in this day and age, but they caught me, and now I'm on a ship with real criminals, murderers, rapists … you name it. It's horrible and I don't deserve this! I try telling them, but they don't care. They're calling me (breaking down in tears again)… an example.

SK: Still surrounded by light, fast forward to the next most significant event in that life in the 1700s and be there now. Notice what's happening.

Haley: I'm in the bottom of a wooden ship. The smell is horrible. There's not enough food. I'm sick with a fever.

SK: Surrounded still by that loving light, go to the last day of your life in the 1700s. Be there now and notice what's happening.

Haley: I slip away and die of fever. I never made it to wherever we were going.

SK: Go ahead and do that now. Find yourself slipping away and floating up into that peaceful space in between lives. Allow a healing, loving light to wash over those events in the 1700s, healing all, washing away your fears. What lessons did you learn in the 1700s?

Haley: You can make plans but sometimes things don't work out.

SK: How is that life affecting you now?

Haley: I'm blessed. I have a good life. I'm afraid of the ship because of my experience, even though we stayed in the lap of luxury with more than enough to eat, amazing accommodations. Hey, I just realized . . . this is a payback of some kind—a reward for what I went through back then, and I should not see it as a punishment.

SK: Nice. Thinking back to the people you knew before and during your trip on the ship in the 1700s, was there anyone there who you know in this current life, yes or no?

Haley: No, but it's still a reward.

SK: Does that mean you're ready to release your fear of ships and enjoy them in your current life?

Haley: Yes.

SK: When would you like to do that?

Haley: Now.

SK: Great, go ahead and imagine an energetic cord connecting you with that ship from the 1700s, and when I count down from three, your spirit guide will cut the cord and you will be free. Three, two, one, cutting that cord. Notice a beautiful bright light is coming down from above, lightening all and healing you and everyone there, totally disconnecting you with that energy. Next, travel to your future in your current life to an event in your future where you have successfully overcome your fear of ships. Be there now. What's happening?

Haley: I'm in the ship. It's far nicer than the last one, and my husband and I are floating around the Greek Isles. It's absolutely gorgeous here and we're having a wonderful time.

SK: Do you feel afraid?

Haley: No.

SK: Not even for a minute?

Haley: I felt a little uneasy when I first boarded and for the first day, but the sea is calm and the food and everything is so nice, I got through it; so after that first evening, I'm good to go. We love our vacation so much, I want to go cruising again.

I absolutely love cruising and discovered my deep resonance with ships originated in several of my past lives, so of course I insisted Haley keep in touch. She and her husband went to Greece and she reported that just as she had foreseen, after some initial apprehension, she had an amazing time. Haley is another example of how you can change your life with just one new decision. Isn't that amazing?

Joanne's Vacation Aggravated a Civil War Trauma

Earlier I mentioned *Supretrovie*, the phenomenon of externally induced past life memories, where souls react to places they've been in past lives. Joanne experienced *Supretrovie* and came to see me after her husband insisted the family spend the summer up near Gettysburg to attend a Civil War reenactment. While there, Joanne felt she had been there in a prior life. Once she returned home, she had unending nightmares and a stabbing pain in her arm that made even simple movement difficult. She went to doctors, but they couldn't find anything physically wrong with her, and even her own husband began accusing her of being a hypochondriac.

During the regression, Joanne experienced herself as a female caregiver to the wounded during the Civil War, somewhere not too far from the Gettysburg site. While she was dressing wounds of the fallen soldiers, the unthinkable happened.

Joanne: I'm on my hands and knees, bending down over a man who has several bullet wounds. He's in bad shape. I'm stuffing the holes as fast as I can, wrapping cloth around his limbs to keep him from bleeding out. I hear a blast from behind me. It's closer than I'd like. The pain is piercing through my upper arm. I've been shot.

SK: Imagine you can breathe and notice a beam of pure white light coming into your arm, healing and relieving you, and you can easily notice who shot you, and what happens next.

Joanne: I can't see. I'm falling over. Blood's everywhere. I'm trying to stop the bleeding by wrapping my apron around my arm, but I'm losing so much blood, I'm dizzy and fall to the ground. I look up and see a man standing over me with a gun. He shoots me and the man I was helping and we're finished.

SK: Still surrounded by that loving, healing light, imagine you can go ahead now and float out of that body, out of that life, and go into the peaceful space in between lives. Imagine the woman who you were back then floats up to speak to you. Notice an energetic cord connecting the two of you and ask her if it would be okay for you to cut that cord now so your arm pain can be healed.

Joanne: Yes, she says that's fine.

SK: Great. Imagine when I count down from three the cord will be cut. Ready? Three, two, one, and cut! A beautiful beam of light is coming through those cords and goes straight into your arm and the arm of the woman you used to be, healing, releasing, and flowing into any other wounds you received during this incident. That light is getting lighter and lighter, brighter and brighter. Let me know when this feels better.

Joanne: (after a couple minutes) It's much better, yes.

SK: Great! Now imagine you can float out into your future in your current life to a moment in your future where you are no longer troubled by this pain in your arm. Be there now and tell me what's happening. What year is this, the first thing that comes to your mind?

Joanne: A few years from now.

SK: Very good. What's happening?

Joanne: I'm actually playing tennis with my daughter. I hadn't been able to play even though I used to enjoy it when I was younger.

SK: Great! How do you feel?

Joanne: So happy and alive. I'm able to move better than I have in a long time.

Once Joanne recognized and healed the true source of her difficulty, her phantom pain from the old arm injury thankfully became a thing of the past.

PTSD—Post-traumatic Stress Disorder

Speaking of war memories from past lives, post-traumatic stress disorder is currently a popular topic in the news. Sadly, with all the military skirmishes around the world, combined with the increase of mass shootings, victims of this very real and debilitating disorder are growing in number.

Post-traumatic stress disorder is a complex diagnosis with several criteria. According to the DSM-5, individuals who have PTSD have been exposed to "death, threatened death, actual or threatened serious injury or actual or threatened sexual violence through direct exposure, witnessing the trauma, learning that a relative or close friend was exposed to a trauma, or had indirect exposure to trauma as in the case of first responders. The individual must also have at least one of the following: nightmares, flashbacks, unwanted upsetting memories, or emotional distress."

I could write a whole book on post-traumatic stress cases alone, but for now, let's take a look at some of my more memorable studies to give you an example of how the RELIEF Method can alleviate such traumas and help people get back to a positive, normal existence.

Because of the wonders of modern medicine, many soldiers survive the battlefields only to return home with unseen wounds. The trauma is often harder to deal with than any physical injury. Emotional scars of witnessing horrors of war can last a lifetime—or as you'll see with these next stories—*lifetimes.*

Natalie Experienced PTSD—from Another Life

Is it possible for someone to still suffer from post-traumatic stress disorder carried over from a past life? During my session with Natalie, I realized that was possible once she told me about the tremendous suffering she had experienced on a trip to Mexico City. Natalie had no idea what caused her to have such bad feelings, but clearly the trip disturbed her deeply.

"I went on a land vacation where we had to fly into Mexico City and spend a couple of nights downtown before going to Oaxaca and some of the other cities," she explained. "I'll never forget that we toured those huge pyramids north of town, and that night, when I came back to my hotel, I started having dreams, or I should say nightmares, of being tied up and burned alive, and I woke up screaming. My friend didn't know what to think. The dreams continued while we were there and I felt better once we got out of the city, but every so often, I still have the dreams. I've always wondered what that was from."

In my research on *Supretrovie*, I realized that you don't have to be on the battlefield itself to have traumatic memories surface.

By the time Natalie came to see me, she had dealt with this issue for years and assumed nothing could be done about it. Once we started talking, she realized there might be a chance to heal her trauma and put an end to her nightmares from what she assumed was a past life. Here's what happened.

> *SK:* Go back to the source event, the very first time you had the experience of being near the pyramids in Mexico. Be there now. Notice what's happening. What year is this?
>
> *Natalie:* 1500s?
>
> *SK:* Are you male or female?
>
> *Natalie:* Female.
>
> *SK:* Alone or with other people?
>
> *Natalie:* Alone.

When people first step into their past lives, they are normally alone, and I typically have to guide them to find memories with other people to uncover the true source of difficulties.

SK: Fast forward to the next most significant event where you are with other people, to the event that causes your nightmares, and be there now. You are surrounded by light, safe and secure. Notice what's happening.

Natalie: I'm alone at first, and things are quiet—too quiet. I went inside a room in that huge temple complex there. It's nighttime and suddenly out of nowhere, I hear shouting and loud booms. I run out to see what's going on and they capture me!

SK: Who?

Natalie: I don't know. Men all in uniforms. They're dragging us away and tying everyone up, setting fire to everything.

SK: Did they mean to kill you?

Natalie: I don't think they set out to, but now that they're here, they don't care. They want domination. That's it.

SK: Allow a bright light to surround you and those events. Lift up out of that scene and float over that life. Imagine the light is healing everything, the sounds and feelings fade away until everything becomes peaceful. Let me know when this feels better.

Natalie: (after a moment) Okay. It's better.

SK: Imagine a cord of light connecting you with those events. Are you ready to cut the cord and free yourself from these memories?

Natalie: Yes.

SK: Very good. Cut those cords. A bright light moves through that cut cord, into your heart, your stomach, your lungs, into your arms and legs and your mind. Allow the light to heal you and remind you that you are no longer connected to the events in the 1500s. Let me know when you feel better.

Natalie: Yes, better.

SK: When will you be ready to completely stop having these nightmares?

Natalie: Now.

SK: Good job. So, what lessons did you learn in the 1500s?

Natalie: Sometimes things are out of your control.

SK: How does that apply to your current life?

Natalie: The company I've worked for the past twenty years recently got taken over and lots of people got laid off, but they kept me. There's still a feeling in the back of my mind that I'll be next and they'll take me out.

SK: Was there anyone you noticed in the 1500s who looked or felt like people you know in your current life?

Natalie: No, but it does make me think that it's a really similar feeling, like you're going to be whacked at a moment's notice. I have to remember that if that does happen, I will be okay.

Natalie's story is a great example that it's not always the *people* from our past who cause our current anxieties, but the *feelings* from prior events that are triggered when we encounter similar challenges in our current lifetime. Once she recognized the similarities in how she felt both in the past and now, Natalie easily released her trauma and moved forward in her life.

I heard from Natalie a couple of weeks after our session and she reported that she hadn't had any nightmares since and felt better than she did before our session.

Doug Had a Case of War Hero Envy

Doug struggled coming to terms with the fact that he did not volunteer for military duty and go to war during his current life; he gained a new perspective after his regression.

"My older brother enlisted in the army against my parents' wishes and went to Iraq back in 2003. He was injured, not seriously, but he damaged his leg enough that he got sent home. I wanted to enlist, too, but my parents couldn't stand the thought of having two sons at war, so I never did and I always felt kind of guilty about that. Guilty and jealous... once my brother came home, I began having strange dreams about battlefields, and all these years later, I never got over them."

Doug explained his nightmares happened at least once a month and when I asked him what he might be doing to bring them on, he couldn't come up with any particular reason. I thought he might be one of those men who love to watch war shows on television, but Doug claimed he rarely watched TV. Still, something clearly troubled him. To his surprise, Doug traveled to a prior lifetime where things were much different.

SK: What year is this, the first thing that comes to your mind?

Doug: 1917.

SK: What's happening?

Doug: I just turned twenty-one and I was drafted into the army. My parents are really upset. I have a younger brother. Wait! He's my older brother now.

SK: Travel to the very last day of your life in the early 1900s and notice how it is that you pass away.

Doug: I was shot. I never made it home. I don't know for sure because I wasn't there anymore, but I don't sense that my brother went to war at all in that life.

SK: How is that affecting your current life?

Doug: We have the opposite going on now. He went to war, I didn't.

SK: When you think about your time in World War I, do those memories cause your nightmares now?

Doug: Oh yes, definitely.

SK: Remember that you are still surrounded by a protective white light, safe and secure, and only that which is of your highest good can come through. Go ahead and go into one of the scenes you find most troubling, only this time, imagine you can float above the event and look down on it. Let me know when you're there.

Doug: I'm there.

SK: Very good. What's happening?

Doug: We're lying on the ground in ditches. There's gunfire all around. Lots of guys are hit and they're moaning and dying all around me.

SK: Very good. Imagine your angel is going to send a huge healing light down on those events and the light is making everything lighter and brighter. The sounds are getting softer and a sense of peace moves over this scene. Let me know when it feels better.

Doug: Yes.

SK: Very good. Now I want you to notice that there is an energetic cord that is coming out of your solar plexus area connecting you with these events. In a moment when I count down from three, your angel will cut that cord and release you. Three, two, one, cutting that cord.

Doug cut cords, and then we did another exercise.

SK: Notice that the soldier who you were then can come out and talk to you now. Imagine he wants you to know that you do not have to continue to relive these events. Have a conversation with him now and let me know what happens.

Doug: He's saying it's okay. I don't need to feel bad for not enlisting this time. I did my duty.

SK: Good job. Now invite your younger brother from that life and your older brother from your current life to join you. Imagine all of you can have a conversation about the lessons that you've come here to learn about as souls. What do they say?

Doug: We're meant to be together. We've been together a lot of other times too.

SK: How many times?

Doug: Four comes to mind.

SK: Good. Any other wars? Imagine you can notice now where you've known each other before.

Doug: One seems like a farm. Not sure when. The other... really ancient. Europe, maybe.

SK: What was your relationship in those lives?

Doug: Same. Brothers. We've always been brothers. In the earlier times we were there for each other. Like we are now. The life in World War I was different. He's saying he never got over it.

SK: What lessons are the two of you learning about together over the course of many, many lifetimes?

Doug: Loyalty. Having someone's back.

SK: Very good. So, is it necessary for you to continue to relive these events from the past?

Doug: No. Not at all. I'm just glad he…(choking up) made it back this time.

SK: Very good.

Once Doug found out that the true source of his guilt and jealousy involved his own post-traumatic stress from times long ago, the unwarranted feelings disappeared. He came to one of my classes a couple years later and reminded me of the session: "My whole outlook changed and my relationship with my brother has never been better."

Helping to heal wounds from past relationships is one of the greatest gifts a past life regression can provide.

Bradley Had PTSD from an Atlantean Disaster

My client Bradley was a successful general contractor in Dallas, Texas. There is a theory that many of the fallen Atlanteans live in the Dallas area and have returned as a soul group to work out their karma together.

Greed and rampant materialism were among the many reasons for the downfall of Atlantis and some of those reincarnated souls came back this time around as materialistic as ever, in order to hopefully grow out of those tendencies and evolve toward more spiritual ideals, ultimately so our planet will avoid another catastrophe.

Bradley came to see me because he'd been dabbling in the metaphysical arena searching for answers about the source of secret panic attacks he'd been suffering from for the past few years. He managed to hide his emotional turmoil from everyone around him, but the attacks started catching up with him.

"When I'm out on site and we're working on imploding old buildings and structures, a horrible fear takes over. My stomach tightens up, I start to sweat. It's awful, and it's only getting worse over time. I try to close my eyes and meditate for a couple minutes, and that worked for a while, but now it's getting worse. I don't know what to do."

Bradley explained that his company demolished older structures all the time.

"It's so hot in summers here, that I'm usually outside when this happens, so people assume I am overheated from the sun, but on the inside, I'm fighting to stand still. There's a deep urge to run far, far away, every time I hear those booming sounds of buildings falling."

I guided Bradley into his past, asking him to travel back in time to the earliest event where this fear of the sounds first began. We soon realized the source of his trouble was earlier than we initially imagined.

SK: Where are you and what's happening?

Bradley: I'm on an island in the ocean.

SK: When is this?

Bradley: Very early. There's no dating system yet. I want to say this is Atlantis.

SK: Very good. What is your purpose in that life?

Bradley: I am an engineer ... well, not an electrical engineer, but structural. I am designing buildings and making sure they can stand up to the high tides and waves. I use special advanced equipment, far beyond anything we have now, to help me build things properly.

SK: Fast forward in time to the events that are causing your current difficulties and be there now. Notice you are still surrounded by healing light and that only that which is of your highest good can come through. Where are you?

Bradley: There's an earthquake. Buildings are crumbling into tiny crumblike fragments. People are screaming, getting crushed.

SK: Did you expect to see your designs fail?

Bradley: No, not at all. If the ocean had risen, the buildings would still remain, but something else is at work. There's a technological cause. Something is disintegrating the buildings and making everything turn into crumbs. It would be like eating a piece of cake, cutting a bite off with your fork and watching as it tumbles down to the plate and turns into crumbs. That sounds strange, I know, but that's what this looks like. Whatever this machine is they've created, it gets inside things and tears the molecular structure completely apart.

SK: Fast forward to the very last day of your life in Atlantis. Be there now. Notice what's happening.

Bradley: I'm falling into the water and getting crushed. Luckily, I wasn't alive by the time that happened. I had already drowned.

SK: Travel up into that beautiful space in between lives and be there now. What lessons did you learn during your time in Atlantis?

Bradley: You can make all the plans you want, but in the end, we are not in control.

SK: How did your time in Atlantis prepare you for your current life? What skills are you using now that you had back then?

Bradley: No doubt, I came to help design new things. Our firm wins awards for ingenuity, but we don't have the ability we did back then, that's for sure. I enjoy what I do, though. It's definitely a talent I have and building is my purpose.

SK: Can you see now where your fear comes from?

Bradley: Definitely.

SK: Would you be able and willing to cut the cords with those past times so you could go out to your jobsites feeling more at ease from this point forward?

Bradley: Yes and no. I can let it go now that I remember, but I always want to keep in mind that we are not in charge. I need to remember so I'll be prepared for what's coming if we don't start doing better this time around. I get a real feeling that we have some major lessons to learn, and if we don't, we're headed for disaster.

In the end, Bradley received his healing, along with a helpful reminder about what is and is not important in life. From then on, he never again panicked at work, or so he said the last time we spoke. I hope his healing continued.

Summing Up

When you think about it, all past life regression involves a story you discover about yourself. It's irrelevant whether that past is on Earth or another planet, from a few years ago or before recorded history. Once you rewrite your back story by healing, releasing, forgiving, and accepting, a new, happier ending is sure to follow. Trauma can devastate your life and make visualizing a bright future next to impossible, but as these clients have demonstrated, there is a light at the end of the tunnel.

CHAPTER 7
....
Vows & Soul Contracts

ONE OF MY FAVORITE ways to work with past life regression is by helping people clear vows and finish up old business of soul contracts they agreed to many lifetimes ago. Believe it or not, this can be a huge source of anxiety for people. By *vows*, I'm talking about saying something like, "I'll never love again!" or "I will be forever in your debt!"

Some vows are more serious than others, obviously, but you get the idea. Souls make vows all the time. When we make such proclamations, we set the wheels in motion for upcoming events and future karma without even realizing what we're doing.

Imagine the havoc you could wreak on your life if you inadvertently agreed to something a thousand years ago and had no idea that decision negatively impacted your current life. By journeying to the source of such events, old agreements can be amended or disbanded altogether so you can move forward. Let's look at some examples of vows and contracts that wreaked havoc on the folks who made them.

Vows

One of the many definitions of a vow is "a solemn promise made to a deity or saint committing oneself to an act, service, or condition."[7]

The entry also cites the origins of the term *vow* and traces that back to Middle English sometime between 1250 and 1300. Can you possibly imagine how many vows we might have entered into since those early days? These next clients got to see firsthand the depths of those solemn promises as they searched for answers about their current lives.

Claudia Vowed to Care for Cats

Earlier in the book, I mentioned Claudia, who moved to her current town to start anew after undergoing counseling for animal hoarding. Hoarding proved to be a past life issue Claudia carried into her current life, but she had another, deeper issue to address.

Claudia's story is a perfect example of how a well-meaning vow wreaks havoc on the current incarnation. Thanks to a court order, Claudia vowed to never take in animals herself ever again and shifted her focus from housing to fundraising. During her regression, Claudia discovered her past life membership in the Bastet cult in ancient Egypt. Her current-life legal agreement to avoid cats directly conflicted with her vow from Egypt. Her commitment to honoring her word impressed me, but unfortunately, at a soul level, Claudia felt miserable. Here's what happened during the rest of her session:

> *SK:* Go back into your life in Egypt, be there now and go to the moment when you are first initiated into the Bastet cult. Let me know when you're there.
>
> *Claudia:* I'm there.
>
> *SK:* Good job. Go ahead and notice yourself and the other initiates taking your vows. Describe this to me.
>
> *Claudia:* There is a High Priestess who is going to each of us and performing a sacred ritual with cleansing and smoke. Then we take our vows.

---

7. "Vow," Dictionary.com. https://www.dictionary.com/browse/vow.

SK: Describe the vows. What were they?

Claudia: In order to fulfill my duties, I vowed to care for cats no matter what, for as long as I live.

SK: Good. Imagine the person you are now, your Higher Self, can go speak to this priestess. Tell her now about all you've done in your current life to help the cats, and ask her if it would be okay to be freed of your vow, as long as you can continue to help the cats by supporting the organizations that protect them. Take your time and see if you can come to an agreement with her.

After a few minutes, sure enough, Claudia made an agreement with the Priestess to end her vow and received cosmic congratulations on her work. She agreed to continue to help animals, but not at all costs. She decided after thousands of years of service, she could relinquish her duties and release the old energy. Next, Claudia ventured into her current-life future, where she visited a future memory.

Claudia: I am now Chairman of the Board of the local chapter of our Humane Society, still busy pulling in funding for the animals. The difference is that I honor myself, I have a peaceful home with one cat and one dog and no desire for more. I do my best to help others care for the animals and I still play my part, but the urgent feeling that caused me so much anxiety over the years, that life-or-death feeling that I have to do this or else, is gone. I feel so much better!

From what I've heard as of our last conversation, Claudia continues her amazing work and now lives a more balanced life after releasing her vows. Claudia's story is a great reminder to leave the past behind and move forward in life. Her tremendous courage to own up to her mistakes is inspired, and shows that with a few internal shifts, you can go on to greatness.

Josh Took His Vow of Silence Too Far

There is a childhood disorder listed in the DSM-5 called *selective mutism* where children have an inability to speak in certain circumstances. You may wonder how this could relate to past lives. My adult clients often recall childhood memories during their regressions. At the age of forty-three, Josh found himself unable to get ahead in his life or career.

Josh grew up in the church, went to Catholic school, and left the religion as an adult. He decided to have a session because he said he didn't feel like he had accomplished anything of great worth. "I guess you could say I'm having a real mid-life crisis. I need to know my purpose and what's holding me back from doing more."

He traveled back in time, and had a big surprise.

SK: Where are you?

Josh: Rome.

SK: What year is this? The first thing that comes into your mind.

Josh: 1362.

SK: Very good. Are you a man or woman?

Josh: A man. I'm a cardinal.

SK: What's happening in 1362 Rome during your life as a cardinal?

Josh: Right now, I see us all gathered together in a room. It's a conclave. We have to elect a new pope. We're in deep prayer in between discussions and committed to listening most of the time to better hear the voice of the Father, of God. We are asking God to guide us in making the right decision. It's so important. It's intimidating.

SK: How is that life affecting you now?

Josh: I have a tendency to listen to others but not offer any of my own opinions. I go along with the group just like I did then.

SK: Theoretically, there's nothing wrong with that, you know?

Josh: Yes, but in modern times, if you don't speak up, nobody notices you. Things aren't like they were back then.

After the fact, I did some research and discovered a conclave convened in 1362 from September 22 through October 28 that resulted in the election of Guillaume de Grimoard as Pope Urban V. According to the Vatican, the number 1362 is an important reference number regarding the Sacrament of the Eucharist:

The sacrificial Memorial of Christ & of His Body, the Church

1362: The Eucharist is the memorial of Christ's Passover, the making present and the sacramental offering of his unique sacrifice, in the liturgy of the Church which is his Body.[8]

Based on this, skeptics might assume this devout Catholic simply recited his scholarship, but is it also possible Josh lived a prior incarnation as one of the twenty cardinals present at the 1362 conclave? I say yes, of course, but it doesn't matter whether or not Josh served as a cardinal so long as he received healing and insight into his current-life dilemma. Here's what happened:

SK: Was your life in Rome the source event of your current life challenges? Yes or no?

Josh: No.

SK: Go to the source event, be there now, and tell me what's happening. What year is this? The first thing that comes to your mind.

Josh: Early, very early.

SK: BC or AD?

Josh: BC, definitely.

SK: Where are you?

Josh: In a school with several people. I want to say this is Greece.

SK: Very good. Are you a man or woman?

Josh: I'm a man.

SK: How do you feel?

Josh: Like I'm part of something bigger than myself. I'm in a group. We all dress alike. We're fighting moral battles with rulers. We have strict rules ... silence.

· · · · · · · · · · · · ·

8. *Catechism of the Catholic Church Part 2: The Celebration of the Christian Mystery Article 3: The Sacrament of the Eucharist.* http://www.vatican.va/archive/ccc_css/archive/catechism/p2s2c1a3.htm.

He flinched a little and looked uncomfortable.

SK: What's happening now?

Josh: I was talking, and I've been asked to be silent. Everyone in the group stops talking except for the leader himself.

SK: How do you feel about that?

Josh: Upset. I came here to be heard and to help change things, so at first, I don't like it. Then I finally give in. It's for a good cause.

SK: How is that affecting you now?

Josh: Same thing. I just learned to be quiet and I get stomped on.

SK: Was your life in Greece the source event of these difficulties?

Josh: No.

SK: Go now to the source event of your difficulties in communicating and be there now. Where are you?

Josh: Asia ... Japan ... China ... Lots of lives there.

SK: What time period?

Josh: So early ...

SK: What was your role in these lives in Asia?

Josh: I was a monk a lot of the time. We constantly fasted and practiced a vow of silence.

SK: How do you feel about being silent during those times?

Josh: Then it was different. I gladly observed silence because it was part of my spiritual practice, a more solitary practice. I didn't feel like controlling people forced me into it.

SK: How are these lifetimes affecting your current life?

Josh: I haven't been able to speak up for myself. I don't want to be greedy, but I should at least say something so I can get what I deserve. When I don't speak, I miss opportunities.

When Josh came out of the trance we talked more about his religion. He was raised Catholic in his current life, and although he said he had a perfectly normal upbringing, as a kid, he had a hard time speaking around priests. Some Catholic denominations observe silence, although the practice is uncommon. Once Josh reached his late teens, he said the uncomfortable feeling went away for the most part, although on the inside, he still felt awkward speaking around them.

The other challenge Josh faced, potentially thanks to so many lives lived in poverty, is his strange relationship with money and inability to accumulate wealth. He was concerned about the current status of his savings and worried he might not have enough to ever retire. We did a healing on his issue with money and worthiness.

> *SK:* Did you, at some time in the past, make a vow of poverty?
>
> *Josh:* Yes, several times.
>
> *SK:* Very good. Imagine you can speak to your former selves. Invite them to be with you today. Notice that many of them lived in poverty because of their religious beliefs. Would it be okay to be complete and release the vow of poverty you took in all prior lifetimes?
>
> *Josh:* Yes.
>
> *SK:* When are you ready to release this vow and accept abundance and prosperity into your life?
>
> *Josh:* Uh … now?
>
> *SK:* Now?
>
> *Josh:* Yeah, now.
>
> *SK:* Very good. Imagine there is a cord of light connecting your current self with all the people you've been before. Bless them and release them as that cord is cut. Notice a bright healing light is coming down from above and moving through you, completely releasing you from the vows you took so long ago.

Next, Josh journeyed into his current-life future. As it turned out, he had a job interview for a much higher-paying position the following week.

SK: Where are you now?

Josh: I had a great interview and I feel good.

SK: Nice! Imagine you can go out further into your future to see how this turned out and be there now.

Josh: I get the job. I'm in my new office and I feel so good. I asked for what I wanted and I'm finally making more money. I feel like I'm getting what I deserve.

Another interesting note about vows and contracts is the fact that I typically avoid any leading questions while doing regression work and attempt to be helpful but vague enough so the client can discover information on their own. Clearing vows is often an exception. In Josh's case, I had to know if his soul made a vow of poverty. Intuitively, I believed he had since he reported many lifetimes living as a monk or priest. I do that because once the person acknowledges the vow exists, they can step into their power by revoking the soul agreement.

Similarly, when I ask clients if they recognize anyone from their current lifetime, they can always say no and that's fine. Despite my intuition, the possibility existed that Josh hadn't made any vows, yet we would still need to clear issues around money and help him come to a new decision in order to create a new result, which is exactly what Josh did. After our session, Josh followed up to let me know he got the job and believed the regression helped him find his voice. As a result, he accomplished something valuable.

Tiffany Vowed to Avoid Having Kids

Recently married in her thirties, Tiffany expressed a deathly fear of pregnancy but had no logical reason for her feelings. "I want my husband to be happy, but when I think of getting pregnant, I start shaking, like I'm having a panic attack. I start sweating, my heart beats out of my chest. It's crazy because there's no reason for this to be happening."

She traveled back in time and relayed the following:

Tiffany: I live near Sedona in the 1800s. I'm a woman and my father is the same father I have in my current life. He was the chief of the tribe and married me off to a very prestigious warrior. I get pregnant and everyone is very happy about that. The tribe gets along well. My father is also the medicine man. We do healings on people and help everyone we can.

Everything sounded wonderful until the situation changed.

SK: Fast forward to the last day of your life in the tribe near Sedona and be there now. Notice how it is you pass into spirit.

Tiffany: I die in childbirth.

SK: Go ahead and float into that peaceful space in between lives, safe and secure, and notice the lessons you learned in that life in the Sedona area. How is that experience affecting you now?

Tiffany: When I realized I wasn't going to make it, I made a vow there and then that I would never have kids.

Not everyone wants to have kids, which is fine, unless she wanted children in her current life and the vow kept her from doing so. She could certainly keep the vow if she liked, but her new husband wanted to have kids soon.

SK: Would you like to clear the vow?

Tiffany: I would, yes.

SK: Was this the first time your soul ever vowed not to have children?

Tiffany: No.

SK: Go back to the source event. Be there now.

Tiffany: I'm somewhere in Europe. Like medieval times. Everyone's sick and dying. The conditions are horrible.

SK: Are you a man or woman?

Tiffany: I'm a man.

SK: How is that life affecting your current situation?

Tiffany: I had a family—a wife and a few kids, but they all died and I'm alone. The world is too horrible to bring anyone else into it, so I make a decision not to have any more kids.

SK: Imagine a bright, healing light, healing and relieving you from your grief. Invite the man who you were back then to come and speak with you now. Tell him that times have changed, and this is a much more sanitary and conducive environment for children. Ask him if it would be okay to change his decision for the future.

Tiffany: Yes, he says that would be okay.

SK: Imagine you can also invite the Native American woman to join you. Imagine a healing light is washing over her pain and ask her if you have permission to have children now. Tell her the same thing.

Tiffany: Yes, she says it's okay.

SK: Very good. Notice if these are the only two times your soul has vowed not to have children. Is it? Yes or no?

Tiffany: Yes.

SK: Very good. Are you ready and willing to break the vow?

Tiffany: Yes.

SK: Let's cut the cords with these two people. Do that now. Imagine a healing light surrounds everyone and let me know when you all feel better.

Tiffany: Yes, it's much better now.

SK: Good. Next, travel to your future in your current life to a time where you are certain you have successfully broken your vow to not have children. Be there now. Notice what's happening.

Tiffany: It's two years from now. I am holding my baby girl. She's healthy, so am I, and we are all happy. Especially my husband. He's thrilled.

SK: How do you feel?

Tiffany: I'm in love with her. She is the best thing I've ever done.

SK: Was it worth it?

Tiffany: Oh yes.

SK: And how did you do physically, having her?

Tiffany: Thanks to modern medicine, everything was relatively easy.

SK: Will you have more children?

Tiffany: Yes, definitely.

Incredibly, I ran into Tiffany a few years later, pushing her little baby girl in a stroller. She seemed quite happy. Had she not wanted children in her current life, then it would not be prudent to clear the vow. Everyone has free will to determine what they choose to experience in life. During the session, she made it abundantly clear that she shared her new husband's wishes to have a baby, and in the end, she did just that.

Derek Suffered from Alien Anxiety

Derek claimed he had been plagued for years with alien visitations that caused him to feel exhausted and tortured. We dove into a session to find out the source of his issues.

SK: Travel back to a time before your current life. Be there now and tell me what's going on.

Derek: I live somewhere else, a planet, only it's nothing like Earth and not in our solar system.

SK: Are you human?

Derek: No.

SK: Imagine your spirit guide is still with you and brings out a mirror that floats down in front of you. Gaze into that mirror and tell me what you look like.

Derek: Oh my god! I'm one of them! A Zeta!

SK: What is a Zeta?

Derek: Zeta Reticulian! The Greys! I'm one of the Greys who's been visiting me!

SK: Where are you from?

Derek: Zeta Reticuli.

SK: What do you look like?

Derek: Gangly and thin, translucent skin, bulbs for eyes. I'm taller than a lot of the Greys.

SK: Great, what arrangement do you have with the Greys?

Derek: I'm teaching them about humans. They want to learn because they have diseases and many of them are dying. They hope humans can help.

SK: Are you helping? Has anything you've done contributed to their well-being so far?

Derek: No, actually, it hasn't at all. Humans have never really been very beneficial to them. Not as much as the media wants you to think.

SK: If that's the case, why are they still bothering you?

Derek: I'm kind of spying on everyone. I'm submitting data to them.

SK: What kind of data?

Derek: Everything—politics, religion, society, and social stuff. They want to see how we do things.

SK: But aren't they more advanced than we are?

Derek: Yes and no.

SK: Would it be okay to wish them well and end your experimentation?

Derek: Maybe.

SK: Imagine one of the beings, whoever is in charge, can come out and join you and your spirit guide. Imagine you and your guide can speak to this Grey and discuss your contract. Let me know when the Grey is there.

Derek: Yes, it's here now.

SK: Does it seem friendly?

Derek: Non-emotional, but not hostile.

SK: Ask the Grey to tell you how long you've had this contract with them.

Derek: Twelve hundred years comes to mind.

SK: Have you been sending data all that time?

Derek: Yes.

SK: What reason did your soul have for agreeing to do this?

Derek: I thought I was helping my people.

SK: Do you really feel like the Greys are still your people?

Derek: Yes and no, but there's nothing good coming out of it anymore.

SK: Imagine you and your guide could speak to this Grey being and rene-
gotiate the terms of your agreement and let me know what that entails.

Derek: It's saying I always had a choice and I could've canceled this a long
time ago.

SK: Why didn't you?

Derek: I never knew that was possible and I'm telling it that I don't think
that's fair because when I was a kid, I didn't remember doing that.
They should've reminded me.

SK: So, is the Grey willing to release you from the agreement?

Derek: Yes. For now, it says.

SK: So, does that mean you will need to assist these creatures in the future?

Derek: Maybe if I go to a new planet after this one.

SK: Is that what you want to do?

Derek: No.

SK: Then go ahead and tell the Grey that now. Ask if you can be done
now and forever more with the arrangement you made.

Derek: I'm talking to it and he is going to ask.

SK: Let me know when it returns and what it says.

Derek: (after a minute) Yes, I can be done. It says there are plenty of others
who are willing to do this, so I don't have to anymore.

SK: How many?

Derek: Hundreds, thousands.

SK: You mean there are potentially thousands of others here on Earth
willing to transmit data to them, or are you talking about people and
beings from other planets too?

Derek: I don't know about other planets. I'm talking about Earth. There
are lots of other species here on Earth besides humans, you know?
Some of the other species help out with data. Humans too.

SK: Where are these other species on Earth and why aren't we aware of
them?

Derek: They're everywhere, all around us. They're disguised as humans, and they're here to cause chaos on our planet. Everybody blames the Greys for all our trouble, but the Greys aren't the ones causing it.

SK: Who is?

Derek: Too many to name. The Grey says this is not important but it's warning me to be careful out here. Earth is a dangerous place.

SK: So, what lessons did you learn from your time with the Greys?

Derek: Loyalty.

SK: Very good. And how is this affecting your current life?

Derek: Loyalty is good to a point, but when it starts affecting your health to the point you can't function, you have to change.

SK: Are you ready to change?

Derek: Oh, definitely.

SK: Very good. Go ahead and imagine a cord of light connecting you and this Grey. In a moment, when I count down from three, your spirit guide will cut the cord and release you from this contract. Ready? Three, two, one, cutting the cord. Imagine your contract is now void, you are now being reprogrammed with peace, joy, and love that you will carry with you and spread to everyone you meet. Continue to allow that healing light to bring peace and joy to your entire body and send that love and joy to the Grey as well. Thank it for allowing you to be released, wish it well, and imagine, when it's ready, that the Grey is floating away. Take your time and let me know when you're finished.

Derek: (after a few minutes) Okay, the Grey's gone.

SK: Wonderful. How do you feel?

Derek: Better.

SK: Nice! Now imagine you can float out into the future, in this current life, to an event where you are putting all this love and joy and light to good use, feeling happy and peaceful, while helping others. Be there now, notice what's happening.

Derek: It's a year from now. I still have my job and things are going better ever since I started sleeping again. I'm at an event. Like a charity thing. We're feeding some people.

Derek: Very good. How do you feel?

Derek: Happy. I'm doing my best to help other people, and my life's never been better.

You may question the validity of Derek's story. As with all my cases, I cannot say for sure whether the information is true or not, but since he believed aliens had contacted him and he found a source event for his soul agreement, cleared the vow, and discovered a solution to living a happier life, that's what's important. Unfortunately, I haven't heard from Derek again, so I hope his life is filled with the joy and peace he desired.

Matt Vowed to Keep His Wife Safe

Matt had been happily married for fifteen years; however, he soon realized the weight of his wedding vows. Within the past year before coming to see me, he began having extreme anxiety about his wife anytime she left the house to go to her new job.

Unlike most married couples, Matt stayed home to raise their kids while his wife worked as an outside sales representative for a pharmaceutical company. Matt took care of their two boys, ages five and seven, and happily drove them to school and picked them up afterward.

Matt voiced his concerns that his wife may be involved in a car accident or might not be safe in the urban metropolis. At first, she apparently laughed it off, but his constant worry caused her to perceive him as overly possessive. They went to traditional counseling, and as a last resort he came to see me for hypnosis.

Matt grew up with a strict religious background. He realized I specialize in past lives, but didn't believe in reincarnation at all, so I kept that in mind during our session. I also wanted to know if he had ever experienced real abandonment issues in his current life that might be at the root of the issue. We talked about his childhood. "Did you have a parent or other significant adult die or leave when you were young?"

"No," he insisted.

"Did anyone leave, or did you move?"

"We lived in the same town, in the same house, our whole life," he explained. "My parents still live there."

When little children are separated from caregivers, some anxiety is normal. Separation anxiety becomes a disorder when these feelings become extreme. At times, they can carry on into adulthood, and I wondered if that might be at the root of Matt's problem. "Did you ever feel like this before?"

"Never."

Clearly, something else was amiss. But what? Intuitively, I knew it must be tied to a past life. Matt went through the guided imagery process and floated out over his early twenties, his high school years, and all the way back to his early childhood. I asked him to notice anything upsetting or unusual. "Go back to the source of this feeling you have about your wife."

Each time I had him observe various aspects of his current life, he found no logical reason for his feelings. Finally, in frustration, he opened his eyes. "This isn't working."

I agreed. After a break I asked him to try once more. He visited his early childhood again, still not experiencing a thing. Finally, I said, "Allow your subconscious mind to take you back to the source event of this issue."

His breathing deepened and he said, "Oh ..."

SK: Where are you?

Matt: I must be imagining things.

SK: That's perfect. What are you imagining?

Matt: There's a street with cars, only they're ... not modern.

SK: Very good. What do they look like?

Matt: (hesitating a moment) Like a Model T or something. I don't know. They're big. Bigger than me. I'm small. This is weird!

SK: That's okay if it seems strange. Continue to use your imagination. Are you looking out from your own eyes?

Matt: Yes.

SK: Look at your hands. What do they look like?

Matt: Like a child.

SK: Very good. Are you alone or with other people?

Matt: There's a woman in front of me. This sounds weird, but ... she's my mother. She's wearing a long wool coat. She is crossing a street.

He shook his head and became agitated.

SK: What's happening now?

Matt: My mother ... she's hit. A car hit her. She's down. I run to her, but ... (becoming emotional).

After surrounding him with light and having him move above these events, we discussed how his mother's death in the prior lifetime affected him now.

SK: How are these events relating to your current life?

Man: My wife, the mother of my children—I promised to keep her safe.

SK: Very good. What relationship does your wife have with your mother in that other situation?

He wiped tears from his cheeks, so clearly something quite real and emotional had happened. I was still careful not to call it a *past life*, because I wanted Matt to feel comfortable opening up about his feelings.

Matt: I don't know ... I don't understand this vision, but for some reason seeing that mother die in front of me makes me worry about my wife. I made a promise to keep her safe and that's what I have to do. Plus, I don't want my kids to lose their mom like I did, although I don't know where any of this is coming from.

Intuitively I believed Matt's mother from the past might be his wife in his current life; however, since I skirted around that fact, I attempted to do the healing a different way.

SK: Can you see now that these two scenarios are unrelated and your wife is safe?

Matt: Yes.

SK: Imagine you can be that little boy and a beautiful light is coming down over you, relaxing you and making you feel better.

More than likely, Matt had made some kind of vow in his past life to keep his mother safe, and that vow meant that he must now keep all mothers safe, especially the mother of his own children. Had he been more open, I would have loved to probe more to see if the mother in that life was now his current-life wife, but again, I kept those thoughts to myself. Knowing the vow was in play and that there was a connection there, regardless of how Matt identified the connection, was all that mattered. After a few minutes of working with the healing light, Matt calmed down. I had him imagine he could travel into the future where he felt better about his wife's new job.

SK: Imagine you are out in an unspecified moment in your future where you are saying goodbye to your wife as she heads out the door. Be in that event now. How do you feel?

Matt: Relieved. I know she will be all right.

SK: How does she behave knowing you support her?

Matt: I've always supported her and I always will. I want her to be happy and she knows how proud I am of her.

Matt's case study is a great example of the fact that people do not necessarily need to believe in reincarnation in order to benefit from a regression. This case also shows how influenced we can be by our past lives, whether we believe in them or not. Many times when people seek past life answers, they instead only go back as far as their earlier current life memories, often for religious reasons. That's what I expected Matt to do; yet, when he allowed himself to use his imagination in a safe way, he received a far greater healing than he expected and used that information to see his relationship in a new way. I did not hear from Matt again, so I can only hope the session helped once he understood the origin of his anxiety.

Summing Up

Vows are some of the most interesting regressions I do. I am endlessly fascinated by the way our souls make decisions so seemingly casually, only to discover that once we make certain choices, all other aspects of our lives must then conform, and not always in ways we like.

PART THREE

. . . . .

Your RELIEF Method Experience

NEXT, BUILDING ON EVERYTHING you've learned so far, you're going to have an opportunity to experience the RELIEF Method for yourself. You've read several of my case studies now and in this section you will use these steps to create a more peaceful experience in your current lifetime. To refresh your memory, RELIEF stands for the following:

Recognize

Recognize the source of the anxiety or trauma and go back to the point of origin where the event first occurred.

In all case histories you've read, I always take the person back to the source event so the situation can be healed at the point of origin. You're going to do this yourself. Sometimes it takes a while to go all the way back to that source, while at other times you will go there immediately. It all depends on what your Higher Self, spirit guide, and soul are ready to experience.

Eliminate

Eliminate the emotional charge by releasing fear or anxiety around the source event. Once the source event or the place where the trauma occurred is identified, a cord of light is cut between you and whatever is causing your anxiety so you are released from that energy.

Lighten

Lighten the frequency of the energy around a given event using healing and vibrational methods.

Once the cord is cut, a healing light is brought in to either neutralize trauma or bring a calming energy of love and peace to the situation until it no longer feels like something that is causing you anxiety.

Integrate

Integrate the new higher frequency energy into the physical, mental, and spiritual bodies by understanding the learning received from experiences.

Once a healing light begins shifting everything, another aspect to healing is to have an epiphany of sorts as to why something happened. This is where you turn your karma to dharma by taking the negative experience and finding the gift and the learning that can be used to bring wisdom to your soul.

Energize

Energize internal thoughts, learnings, and holographic thoughtforms around the issue so they become incompatible with the lower frequencies of fear, stress, and anxiety.

Once the learning is recognized, an energetic shift occurs so you are able to move forward in life with the new mindset.

Future

Future progress into a scene in the current lifetime where the situation is completely resolved and healed. Bring that energy back to the present day and move on in life with a new perspective.

Once you travel to your current-life future, you will hopefully visit an event where you can experience firsthand how different you feel since your healing. Then you can bring that energy back to today and move forward in your current life in the direction of greater happiness, joy, and peace. Ready to try it?

CHAPTER 8

· · · · · · · · ·

Guided Journeys & Exercises for Positive Change

IN THIS CHAPTER, YOU will have the opportunity to go through a series of progressive exercises, with each one building on the prior, that you can use to loosen your grip on your current circumstances and open yourself up to healing the past and moving into a higher state of being. Hypnotic journeys are a process, not a destination. Remember Carol, who was afraid of tunnels and had to come in for more than one regression to get to the bottom of her issue? Sometimes that's what it takes.

All guided journeys in the book are meant to be experienced in layers so that new insights can come through over time, when your soul and Higher Self are ready to integrate new information. Use these as often as needed to receive your answers. Each time you go through one of the journeys, you will experience peeling back more onion-like layers of memory.

Also, you'll have to get used to doing these processes, which is why each one builds on the last so that it's like working out at the gym, strengthening your muscles more and more each time you exercise. Likewise, each session helps you build more insight and gain new strength to face your future and create the best possible life for yourself, so it's something you can do repeatedly, whenever you'd like.

Speaking of which, in order to get the most out of these exercises, I highly recommend recording yourself and listening to the recordings so you will get the full benefit of the processes.

I understand you may not like the sound of your own voice on a conscious level, but believe me, on a subconscious level, your soul loves to hear you speak.

Making recordings now is easier than ever before. There are several free recording apps you can download to your phone or device, then just read the passages and create your own personalized journeys you can use again and again. With that, let's begin!

Journaling & Letting It All Out

Writing about your experiences can be an important part of releasing your anxiety and relieving trauma. Before I work with clients, I always have them write a letter so the mind can begin working on what needs to heal, and I'd like you to do the same.

I assume if you're reading this, something in your past troubles you. Although you may or may not know where the issue began, I would bet you do know what it feels like, or what difficulties the situation has created in your current life.

Exercise
· · · · · · ·

To help jog your memory, I will guide you through some questions that will help you uncover what you most want to release.

1. Think of things you fear—animals, situations, or people. Make a list of anything that comes to mind, and keep adding on more, whenever you think of something new.

2. Once your list is complete, go through and determine which fears are reasonable and which are beyond what you would consider normal. Circle anything that either really bothers you or that you feel is excessive.

3. Next, for each item you listed, to the best of your ability and recollection, write the cause or source of your fear. For example, if you're afraid of snakes, do you believe that started when you were a child after you almost stepped on one, or does the fear go much deeper? Sometimes we think we know the cause of our anxieties and fears, but often hypnotherapy uncovers more than we initially realized. For the most part, each of us has some idea of why we feel a certain way about the things that consciously bother us.

4. Write down any other difficulties that are troubling you in any of the major areas of your life—love and relationships, your health, or finances and money.

5. Do you suffer from anxiety? If so, when did that start?

6. If and when you do have panic attacks, how do those begin? For example, do you get a tingling feeling and then your head hurts, or what exactly happens when the panic starts? What are you doing when that happens? Maybe you're driving, or at work, or talking to a certain person. Perhaps you never stopped to think of these source issues or triggers before, but bringing some awareness to how and why this happens is incredibly helpful information that will assist you in releasing those energies.

Take your time and write as though you're speaking to your best friend. Nobody will see this but you, so be honest and thorough. Keep your journal handy as you go through the exercises in the rest of the book so you can make notes along the way about thoughts and ideas you want to keep track of later on.

Deep Breathing for Relaxation

I am a big fan of breathing exercises to create calm in the body. One of my favorite places to do this is during my yoga classes. I highly recommend practicing yoga. There is nothing as relaxing and healing as stretching the body while breathing deeply. Your breath connects your mind to your body and can create deep peace that can take the edge off even the most acute stressors.

Aside from the amazing benefits of exercise, one reason yoga is so powerful is the breathing techniques you learn that help you concentrate on becoming consciously aware of your breathing habits, which can be a major contributor to stress and anxiety. The best breathing exercises are simple and designed to bring your conscious awareness to the breath, thereby forcing you to slow down and relax.

Breathing in and out through the nose is most beneficial because it activates the parasympathetic nervous system, which helps the body rest and digest food. Breathing out of the mouth activates the sympathetic nervous system, our fight-or-flight impulses, and actually raises the stress hormone cortisol, blood pressure, and adrenaline.

That makes sense. Back when we lived in caves, we needed extra adrenaline to give us the strength to outrun predators. Mouth breathing would save lives by increasing the hormones that help get us moving in a hurry.

In modern society, running for our lives, charging after our food or sprinting from predators is unnecessary. Consciously stepping back and breathing slowly and fully through the nose allows the lungs to fill evenly, which naturally calms you down.

Studies now show that people prone to anxiety often hyperventilate, just as many of my clients have described to me over the years. This is a direct function of mouth breathing, panicking without the proper tools to calm down. When you begin to pay attention to proper breathing, the body naturally heals itself and goes back to normal functioning, making you feel calm, controlled, and relaxed.

Our yoga instructor instructs us to do the Ujjayi Breath by taking a deep, healing breath in through the nose and exhaling through the nose, while imagining the breath rolling over the back of the throat like a wave in the ocean crashing on the shore. This deep breathing keeps the body warm so the muscles and the nervous system can rest.

Once the Ujjayi breath is established, you can then work on balancing the inhalations and exhalations by counting in your head so that the amount of time you take to inhale is the same as the amount of time you exhale. This also creates balance, and if you're worried about something, the activity gives your mind a simple task to think about so you can release worries and concerns.

While it would be wonderful to take yoga whenever possible, you may not have time, and learning to do simple breathing is something you can do in a couple of minutes each morning before you start your day, before you go to sleep, or any time you need better control of your emotions. Let's do a short exercise so you can try this yourself. You may want to record this section for future use.

Exercise
. . . .

Sit in a comfortable chair with your hands in your lap and feet flat on the floor. Close your eyes and begin to notice your breathing. Take a deep, healing breath in through your nose. Exhale out of your nose.

If you find this difficult to do at first, then breathe in through your nose and exhale out of your mouth. The more you practice, the easier this will get.

Feel the breath going into the body. Imagine you are breathing in love, and joy, and relaxation, and exhaling tensions and stress. Very good.

Notice that with each breath you take, you are beginning to feel lighter and more relaxed.

Next, breathe in through your nose to the count of four. Ready?

Breathing in one … two … three … four … and exhaling one … two … three … four. Balance the inhalations with the exhalations.

Breathing in one, two, three, four; exhale one, two, three, four.

Very good.

And again—breathing in one, two, three, four; exhaling one, two, three, four.

Continue to do this for several minutes. As you do, imagine any tensions in the body begin to disappear. With each full breath you take you will become more and more peaceful and relaxed.

Continue to breathe in peace, joy, and love, one, two, three, four; and exhale tension, one, two, three, four, allowing all tensions to leave the body now. Good job.

Breathe in peace, joy, and love, one, two, three, four; and now exhale peace, joy, and love, one, two, three, four; send positive feelings into the world.

And again, breathe in peace, joy, and love, one, two, three, four; and now exhale peace, joy, and love, one, two, three, four; send love and light into the world.

When you feel fully rested and refreshed, open your eyes and go about your day.

You can do this balanced breathing exercise any time you need to get a little extra energy, and if you would like, you may want to record any thoughts or feelings in your journal. How much better do you feel letting go of unwanted emotions and replacing them with new, loving thoughts? Enjoy the journey and do this process often, whenever you need to feel uplifted.

Progressive Muscle Relaxation

One of the most helpful exercises for people suffering from stress and anxiety is to do progressive muscle relaxation to help take charge and gain control of stress. This will build on what we did a moment ago with the breath; however, this time not only will you concentrate on breathing but you will also focus your mental powers on different muscle groups, tensing them and then consciously releasing the tension.

Muscle relaxation exercises are incredibly effective because you use the power of your conscious mind to willfully become tense and you then choose to release that tension, giving yourself a feeling of control over your own anxiety by commanding tension to leave the body. Let's go ahead and do a simple yet powerful progressive muscle relaxation and you will see for yourself how helpful this can be. Feel free to make a recording if you'd like.

Exercise
. . . .

Sit in a comfortable chair with your hands in your lap and feet flat on the floor. Close your eyes.

Take a deep, healing breath in through your nose. Exhale out of your nose. Feel the breath going into the body. Imagine you are breathing in love, and joy, and relaxation, and exhaling tensions and concerns. Very good.

Breathing in one ... two ... three ... four ... and exhaling one ... two ... three ... four.

Breathing in one, two, three, four; exhaling one, two, three, four. Very good.

With each breath you take, you are becoming more and more relaxed.

Imagine you can focus your attention on your head. Squeeze your eyes and crinkle your nose. Tighten those muscles as tight as you can. Inhale. Hold it, one, two, three, four; then exhale one, two, three, four, and release the tension.

Next, move to your jaw. Tighten your jaw muscles by squeezing your lips and jaw into a big smile. Breathe in as you tighten your jaw and lips. Hold it, and exhale as you release your mouth and jaw. Imagine noticing how much more relaxed your jaw is now.

Next, imagine you can scrunch your shoulders up toward your chin. Breathe in as you tighten your shoulder muscles. Hold it, one, two, three, four; then exhale one, two, three, four, as you release that tension. Very good!

Next, breathe in as you tighten your hands into fists and squeeze the muscles in your arms. Hold it for one, two, three, four; then exhale one, two, three, four as you release that tension. Imagine your arms feel heavy and relaxed.

Now tighten your abs and stomach muscles. Squeeze your stomach as you inhale through your nose. Hold it for one, two, three, four; then exhale for one, two, three, four, as you release all the air from your lungs and feel your stomach muscles relax.

Take a deep breath in while you squeeze your buttocks. Hold it for the count of one, two, three, four; then release and exhale for one, two, three, four.

Breathe in again while you tighten your thigh muscles by squeezing your hamstrings together for one, two, three, four; then exhale for one, two, three, four and release.

Tighten up the muscles in your feet, squeezing your toes and tightening your calves as you inhale for one, two, three, four; then exhale one, two, three, four, and let that go.

Now, to the best of your ability, go ahead and take a deep breath in while you tense up every single muscle in your body. Breathe in and hold that for one, two, three, and four; then release all your muscles in your body while you exhale for one, two, three, and four.

Notice your entire body feels more relaxed than before and notice how easy it is for you to release tension from the body. Good job!

Open your eyes, and go about your day, feeling awake, refreshed, and better than you did before.

How did that feel? Once you consciously begin to tense yourself up and allow tension to leave the body by taking control of your physical stress, it will become easier to do so when things are stressful in your outer world. By deeply breathing and consciously deciding to release tension, your body, mind, and spirit will become more peaceful and serene.

If you feel guided to, you may want to write down in your journal any ideas or thoughts that occurred to you. Often, deep breathing and relaxing your muscles can actually help you let go of painful memories so you can replace them with positive messages of joy and peace. This process only takes a second to do, and yet it is a real game-changer in terms of how you feel and how you determine your emotional outcome for your day ahead and for your life. Good job!

Finding Your Happy Place

We all need a place to call home, even during a past life regression. Several years ago, I created my own version of my Happy Place, and to this day this area serves as a launching pad for all my guided journeys.

Creating a safe space in your mind's eye where you begin your journey helps build your confidence to move into the realm of the unknown.

This next journey will help you discover and travel to your Happy Place, filled with things that make you feel peaceful and at ease. While your Happy Place exists only in your mind's eye, once established, this inner sanctuary becomes quite real. Simply close your eyes and access this space whenever necessary. To give you a better idea of what the Happy Place is like, I received some feedback from one of my clients who shared a vivid description of her own sacred space: "My room is bright pink! Shiny crystals, pink sofas, pink overstuffed chairs—felt like Disneyland! Fun, safe, happy, and filled with safety."

Other clients described cabins in the woods, tiny houses on the beach, and everything in between. What your place is or where it's located doesn't matter. What matters is that you love it and it makes you feel happy and safe. Ready to find your Happy Place? Let's begin!

Exercise

Sit in a comfortable chair with your hands in your lap and feet flat on the floor. Close your eyes.

Take a deep, healing breath in through your nose. Exhale out of your nose. Feel the breath going into the body. Imagine you are breathing in love, and joy, and relaxation, and exhaling tensions and concerns. Very good.

Go ahead and balance your breathing. Notice how you can breathe in for a certain amount of time as you did earlier, and exhale for the same amount of time. Allow your body to relax. You may also breathe in positive feelings and find yourself exhaling any unwanted emotions or energies. Good job!

Allow a beam of pure white light to come down through the top of your head, moving down into your eyes, your nose, your jaw.

Continue to breathe as the light moves down into your neck and shoulders, your arms, elbows, wrists, hands, and fingers, flowing down your spine into your heart, your lungs, toward the base of your spine, flowing down your legs into your feet.

Notice the light pours out of your heart, creating a beautiful golden ball of light that surrounds you by about three feet in all directions. Imagine yourself floating inside this peaceful golden ball of light as you breathe in one, two, three, four, and exhale, one, two, three, four.

Know that within this healing golden light, only that which is of your highest good can come through.

Very good.

Go ahead and imagine there is a doorway in front of you. You can see the door, feel the door, or just have an inner knowing that there is a doorway in front of you.

When I count to three, you will walk through that door. Ready? One, two, three, opening the door.

Open the door now and walk or float inside a beautiful space that you love and enjoy. Feel the wonderful healing energy of your special place as you start to look around. You may notice if you are indoors or outdoors, whether this is a sunny day or a cloudy day, or perhaps you are inside a beautiful room. Take a moment now and go into this place where you feel totally safe, secure, and energized.

By the time I count to three, you will arrive in your Happy Place. One, two, and three, you're there. Be there now and notice how peaceful you feel. Know that this is a special space and you can come here at any time to receive healing.

Take a deep breath in through your nose, one, two, three, four, and exhale one, two, three, four, as you allow yourself to become completely relaxed inside your special Happy Place. Breathe in the energy of joy, peace, and happiness as you inhale one, two, three, four, and exhale one, two, three, four. Very good.

Turn around now and walk back through the door, knowing you will easily be able to return to your Happy Place as many times as you would like to or need to in the future.

Be back where you started. In a moment, when I count down from five, you will come back into the room, feeling awake, refreshed, and better than you did before.

Five—grounded, centered, and balanced

Four—continuing to process this new energy in your dreams tonight so by tomorrow morning, you will be fully integrated into your new Happy Place

Three—still surrounded by that beautiful golden ball of light, knowing that only that which is of your highest good can come through, you will find yourself driving carefully and being careful in all activities

Two—grounded, centered, and balanced, and

One—you're back!

Great job! How did you enjoy discovering your Happy Place? Was it what you expected? What surprised you?

You may want to do some journaling about some of the details of your Happy Place because you will visit your special spot quite a bit in the upcoming processes. Take notes about anything you believe is important. What did it look like? Indoors or outdoors? Journal about the details, as much as you can recall, and know that the space may evolve and change some too. The most important aspect of the Happy Place is that you love being there and can use this as a home base, so to speak, for the rest of your journeys. Good job!

Meeting Your Spirit Guide

One of the most important aspects of hypnotherapy is to enlist the support of a spiritual guide or angel who can act as your facilitator and all-knowing partner. They will remain by your side while you're embarking on your journeys, providing safe passage through the inner workings of your mind.

According to a CBS News poll, roughly eight out of ten Americans believe in angels.[9] Other people prefer to think of these celestial helpers as spirit guides, while others work with animal totems. I've worked with all three during different times in my life. No matter what you call the being who shows up to assist you, having an omnipotent helper can be hugely beneficial.

When you do journey work, aside from locating a special and safe space to work from, such as your Happy Place, there is also an added sense of peace that comes from knowing a trusted friend is by your side—someone who has your back and knows everything there is to know about you. Who better to help you out than a guide who has been with you for potentially millennia or longer?

Here's a description my client Marie gave me about meeting two of her guides: "My Angel met me. She wore white and had long, wavy chestnut hair. She presented me with a bright pink heart. The heart was full of 'authentic love.' She placed the heart energy into my body. My whole body radiated bright pink, loving light. Then I handed the Angel a watch. The watch represented 'time.' I felt a release of keeping time schedules and anything associated with time. A turtle then came to see me. The turtle represented time and sent the message to slow down. I am not supposed to rush but to stay calm and slow down."

In this example, Marie met two of her guides, which is certainly possible. You don't always know for sure who will show up until it's happening. For the intent of our exercises, you only need to connect with one major guide who assists you through the rest of the RELIEF program.

I believe we all have many unseen guides and helpers who work with us during different chapters of our lives, so the guide you meet here may be specifically designed to help you with the issues you will resolve during your RELIEF process. Let's go meet your guide, or if you already know them, this will be a great opportunity to reconnect. Ready? Let's begin!

. . . .

9. Poll: Nearly 8 in 10 Americans believe in angels—CBS News, last modified December 23, 2011. https://www.cbsnews.com/news/poll-nearly-8-in-10-americans-believe-in-angels/

Exercise
· · · · · · ·

Sit in a comfortable space and close your eyes.

Take a deep, healing breath in through your nose. With each breath you become more and more relaxed.

Continue to breathe in peace, joy, and love, one, two, three, four, and exhale tension, one, two, three, four. Good job.

Breathing in peace, joy, and love, one, two, three, four, and now exhaling peace, joy, and love, sending positive feelings into the world.

Very nice! Now bring your beam of pure white light through the top of your head. Allow that light to move into your eyes, your nose, your jaw, into your neck and shoulders, into your arms and down your spine.

Continue to breathe in this loving light as it moves down, down, down, toward the base of your spine, flowing into your thighs, your knees, your calves, your ankles and heels, and down into the soles of your feet and into your toes.

Imagine the light is getting stronger now as it moves from the crown of your head, all the way into your legs and down to the soles of your feet.

Go ahead and create your beautiful golden ball of light that surrounds your body in all directions. Float inside the golden ball of light, feeling safe and secure and knowing within the golden light only that which is of your highest good can come through. Notice a doorway in front of you. You've been here before, so go ahead and walk through that door now. Ready? One, two, three, walking through the door into your Happy Place.

As you start to look around your Happy Place, enjoying yourself, I want you to imagine someone floating down from above and joining you. Notice if this is an angel, a spirit guide, a friend or loved one who has passed into spirit, or some other helper. Very good. Know that from now on we will refer to your special someone as your guide. Imagine your guide is there with you now, and they say hello to you.

Your guide may be someone you've worked with before, or it might be someone new. Either way, say hello and thank your guide for being here today. Notice the deep feeling of unconditional love and high regard your guide has for you. Very good. Your guide is a helper who has been with you for a very, very long time, and who knows every single thing there is to know about you and your soul, and your soul's journey.

Take a few moments to connect with your guide and ask them any questions you'd like. When you're finished, imagine you can thank your guide for being here today and watch as they float up, up, up, back to where they came from. Know that you will see your guide again soon.

Turn around now and walk back through the door, back to where you started.

In a moment, when I count down from five, you will come back into the room, feeling awake, refreshed, and better than you did before.

Five—grounded, centered, and balanced

Four—continuing to process this new energy in your dreams tonight so by tomorrow morning, you will be fully integrated into these new insights

Three—still surrounded by that beautiful golden ball of light, knowing only that which is of your highest good can come through, you will find yourself driving carefully and being careful in all activities

Two—grounded, centered, and balanced, and

One—you're back!

Nice job! Did you enjoy seeing your guide? Was this a divine energy you had worked with before, or someone new?

If you'd like, you may want to take a moment or two to write down anything important your guide shared during this first meeting. There will be more to come, believe me. For now, continue to keep the peaceful feelings of love and contentment with you as we continue on.

Cutting Cords

Throughout the book, I've mentioned cutting cords, which is one of the best processes you can do anytime to relieve stress and anxiety. Cutting cords can be done to release tension between you and anything that causes you stress. The idea is simple—you use your imagination to acknowledge an energetic cord connects you with everyone and everything. If tension needs to be eased, you cut the cord and send a healing light to you and the other person. Cutting cords does not mean we are disconnecting from them forever. Instead, the process is like sending the person a bright blessing. During the processes in the upcoming chapters, you'll be doing a lot of cord-cutting as part of your journeys, but for now, let's try a simple example of how this works.

Exercise
· · · · · · ·

Sit in a comfortable space, close your eyes, and begin to breathe deep, healing breaths. Find yourself feeling relaxed and go ahead and imagine a beautiful ball of golden light surrounding you, protecting and healing you. Very good.

Imagine you are in this safe space and that you can now invite anyone or anything that is bothering you to float out in front of you. This may be a person, such as a boss or coworker or anyone you've had difficulties with in the recent past.

Imagine this is the person's Higher Self, their soul, floating in front of you, so regardless of their behavior in the real world, this is the best version of them who is meeting with you right now. If needed, allow them to apologize to you. If possible, accept that apology and notice there is a cord of light connecting the two of you. The cord may be coming out of your stomach/solar plexus area, connecting you with that other person.

Imagine your guide is appearing with a huge pair of golden scissors. In a moment, when I count to three, your guide will cut the cord. Ready? One, two, three, cutting the cord.

Notice as the cord is cut, a beautiful healing light pours down from above. Moving through that cut in the cord, the light moves into your body, healing and releasing, and it also provides healing to the other person.

Imagine the other person becomes so light and bright that they float away. Good job.

Notice that light continuing to move from your stomach, into your heart, down into your legs and feet and moving up into your mind. You feel lighter and brighter than before.

When you're ready, thank your guide for assisting you today and on the count of three you will return, coming back into the room, feeling awake, refreshed, and better than before.

One—grounded, centered, and balanced; two, continuing to receive healing from the light; and three, you're back!

How did that work for you? How do you feel? Record any thoughts in your journal. I promise you will receive amazing benefits from sending love and blessings to the difficult people in your life. I've seen miracle after miracle over the years doing this process because even though you're working in your mind, the person receives the healing at the soul level.

Clients who have had huge fallouts with a family member they had not spoken to in years found that after cord-cutting they received calls, reconnected, and healed old wounds. You feel better and neutralize the energy around the person and move on with life in a more peaceful way.

With practice, you won't need a whole guided journey to cut cords. Are you having a rough day at work? Spend a moment with your eyes closed and cut cords with the source of your angst. You will often see immediate results. There is a theory that we are all one. I believe that's true. Everyone you meet is a reflection of you, so when you heal the part of you that is reflected in another person by extending them grace, healing, love, and forgiveness, everyone benefits—especially you. By shifting the way you view the other person, you instantly change and receive a new outcome.

Creating Positive Affirmations

Once we set the clear vision for where we want to go and release our past stress and tension, another critical aspect for our success involves monitoring our thoughts to make sure we put only positive supporting material into our minds. Your mind is like a computer, so if you aren't pleased with what you've been getting, the best way to receive better results is by reprogramming yourself. Affirmations and mantras are powerful tools.

I love affirmations—encouraging scripted messages that help reprogram our inner minds so we can achieve optimal results. It's important to come up with some good affirmations you can either say to yourself, write down, post on your mirror to read in the morning before work, or leave in a place where you can see it, wherever that might be.

Affirmations can be created to assist you with any area. To create meaningful messages for yourself, go back and review your journal to see if any ideas pop up.

Affirmations should be written in the affirmative about the state of being you would like to be in rather than where you are at the moment, as if you already have what you want. For example, if you need a better job, you would use an affirmation such as:

I work for a wonderful employer who appreciates me.

You can create affirmations for just about anything you need to improve. For additional income, you could say:

I easily attract money, or *I always have*
more than enough money to meet my needs.

One of my personal favorites that I've used for years on a daily basis is:

I am healthy—body, mind, and spirit.

Theoretically you may not feel well on a day you use the affirmation above, but if you keep saying it with emotion, you will invariably reprogram yourself to what you want. To assist with stress and anxiety, you could craft a simple affirmation such as:

I am calm and relaxed, I am calm and relaxed, I am calm and relaxed.

Repeat the sentiment, combine that with some deep breathing, and feel better. I recommend writing out possible affirmations you can use. What area of your life do you want to work on first? Put your desire in writing, sprinkle it around your home and office, and watch for results.

Here are a few simple steps you can use to create your own positive affirmation:

1. Make a list of areas you would like to see improvement on, such as work, relationships, health, or income. To give you a few ideas, you can also refer back to Chapter One and the section on why people seek regression.

2. Practice writing out positive statements about those items as if you already have them.

3. Recite them aloud. How do they make you feel?

4. Make note of your new affirmations and place them where you will see them.

5. Repeat for thirty days and watch for results or improvements.

One important aspect to consider is the language you use. Make sure your words resonate with your soul and have special meaning so they work better. For example, I might like the word *bliss* and you may prefer to say *harmony*. There are certain words that represent feelings and concepts that have deep meaning for you, so always use what you love.

You can refine these whenever you'd like. Repeating the affirmations for thirty days is important because it takes a period of time to notice real effects. You don't have to take much time with these, either. Once you create affirmations that sound good to you, write them down, and put them someplace you'll see them every day, like on a mirror; then know that whether or not you are consciously focusing on them or not, your subconscious mind, where all lasting change begins, is busy picking up on your desires and creating them in the outer world.

Meditation & Mantras

I meditate daily and highly recommend you do the same. Even after years of doing this, my meditation practice continues to be the best gift I've ever given myself. Sitting still with your eyes closed, even if it's just for a few minutes in the morning and evening, can make a huge impact on lowering your daily stress levels. I've found meditation to be critical for my overall happiness in life and there are hundreds of studies that prove the benefits of taking a little *me time* every day, especially if you're challenged by stress, depression, or anxiety.

The idea of meditation seems daunting because many people have the initial impression that meditation takes tons of time. I promise it doesn't. Close your eyes and do some deep breathing for five minutes in the morning before you start your day and five minutes in the evening, either right after coming home from work or right before you go to bed at night, and you won't believe how much more relaxed you'll feel.

The other misconception about meditation that stops a lot of my clients is the idea that in order to meditate you need to have a completely silent mind. Nothing could be further from the truth. Your mind thinks. That's what it does, and you cannot get your mind to stop thinking. That is not possible. What you can do is give your mind something productive to think about. That's where mantras come in. One of the easiest ways to meditate is to use a *mantra,* or a simple word or phrase, repeated over and over in your mind so that you consciously acknowledge that your mind wants to work and think, and you give your mind something to think about.

Let's say you want to affirm that you are calm and relaxed, so you could use that as your mantra by sitting with your eyes closed and repeating:

I am calm and relaxed, I am calm and relaxed, I am calm and relaxed.

Turning any of your affirmations into reaffirming mantras is a great thing to do, especially if you've taken time to come up with some good affirmations using words and concepts that you love. While phrases can make awesome mantras, most mantras are one word. A great one-word mantra you could recite is the word OM, which you can say to yourself or aloud while breathing and closing your eyes. Repetition is the key to effectively using mantras, because when you allow your mind to focus on a word you love, the mind will be steered away from the unhelpful thoughts causing you stress and anxiety.

Another easy and very effective mantra I've recommended to many of my clients is to repeat your own name either aloud or to yourself, over and over again, as unwanted thoughts leave. As I've told you earlier, just like your subconscious loves to hear your recorded voice, it also loves to hear your name.

While you're repeating your mantra, whatever you've chosen, your conscious mind will slowly begin to let go of negativity and you will start to feel your whole body relax.

Along the lines of some of our earlier exercises, another one I've been using lately is to simply count and balance my breath, using the numbers as a sort of mantra. Let's say I want to inhale to a count of eight. I simply say: one, two, three … and so on while concentrating on my breathing. Then I exhale while saying one, two, three and so on until I exhale to the desired number. I normally say the number mantra silently to myself because a lot of times I'm at the gym walking on a treadmill. That just goes to show, you can meditate just about anywhere. Even concentrating on something as mundane as counting to eight can dramatically improve your overall mindset, aside from the extra oxygen your brain receives when you're breathing properly. Stress has to leave.

Try any of these ideas or repeat any other pleasant words you like such as *joy, peace, love*—anything that resonates with you. Allow your mind to relax. While you breathe, repeat your chosen word and you will feel greater relaxation and inner peace.

Using mantras does not need to take a lot of your time. Even if you redirect your thoughts for a couple minutes each day, the results should speak for themselves.

Summing Up

All the ideas and processes in this book are things I've not only recommended to others but I've done myself to navigate the waters of life. I do many of these practices on a daily basis to help me remain grounded in gratitude and to send blessings to all around me. I hope the ideas work wonders for you! Next up, we will dive deeper by going into some longer guided exercises.

CHAPTER 9

· · · · · · · · · ·

Past Life Clearings

NOW THAT YOU'VE HAD a chance to experience the RELIEF Method through case studies of other people, in this chapter you'll travel back in time to uncover your own source of events that occurred before your birth in your current incarnation.

When you're going into past lives, it's important not to judge yourself, even though that's often easier said than done. What I mean by that is that your first impression when you see an event that occurred hundreds of years ago is to say, "It feels like I'm making this up," or "This seems crazy, or weird."

Even some of my clients, as you read in part two, thought the same thing, and believe it or not, so do I whenever I take a past life journey—*even to this very day!* Especially when I'm working with my students, I often find myself telling them that I am surely making this all up, so don't feel bad if you do the same.

Some of the insights are so out of the realm of your personal experience or conscious thinking that the revelations can be quite surprising; it's natural to feel like you're making it up. But then again, where do you believe this comes from? And what if it is true? What if it's not? As I've said before and I will continue to remind you—it doesn't matter whether this is real or not.

Your personal happiness in your current life is all that matters. So go easy on yourself. Think of this as an amazing adventure you're about to embark on and have some fun with it while seeing what comes up for you.

Speaking of adventure and unexpected outcomes, another situation that might happen is you will travel back in time and only go as far as your current life. If that happens, that's perfectly normal and okay. I've related hypnosis to a good gym workout: Sometimes you need to flex those muscles a little and practice going back to things that happened in your current life before you can return all the way back to some other lifetime. You can always do the journeys again, and over time, with your intentions set to visit your past lives, it will eventually happen. Let's get started!

Clearing Past Life Anger

Over my many years in private practice, I have found that souls express themselves with love on the positive side, and one of two undercurrents of negative emotion—either anger or sadness. Some people, you may notice, have an undercurrent of anger. You can just look at them and see that at any moment, they are about to blow a gasket. Physically, they may have high blood pressure, reddening in the face when they get frustrated, or ball their fists and appear out of breath and exasperated. I'm sure you probably know people like this, right?

Other souls have a mellower way of being. They may get periodically depressed, quiet and sullen, disappear, and only show up when they're in a good mood. These folks likely have a deep undercurrent of sadness. There is an old saying you may have heard that depression is simply *anger turned inward.* The sad person won't want you to notice they're not upbeat, so they turn their feelings inward, and don't let anyone know that things are eating them up from the inside out. They are people pleasers who do not want to offend anyone, and as such, they hide their darker thoughts from others.

Anxiety, depression, and trauma are undoubtedly rooted in anger and sadness. For this reason, it's important to release anger and sadness first before we move on. Know that you are always assisted by your loving spirit guide and that in the end, you will feel lighter than before. Ready? Let's do this!

Exercise

Sit in a comfortable chair with your hands in your lap and feet flat on the floor. Close your eyes.

Take a deep, healing breath in through your nose. Exhale out your nose. Feel the breath going into the body. Imagine you are breathing in love, and joy, and relaxation, and exhaling tensions and concerns. Very good.

Breathing in one ... two ... three ... four ... and exhaling one ... two ... three ... four.

Breathing in one, two, three, four; exhaling one, two, three, four.

Very good.

With each breath you take, you are becoming more and more relaxed.

Continuing to breathe in peace, joy, and love, one, two, three, four, and exhaling tension, one, two, three, four, allowing all tensions to leave the body now. Good job.

Breathing in peace, joy, and love, one, two, three, four, and now exhaling peace, joy, and love, one, two, three, four, sending positive feelings into the world.

And again, breathing in peace, joy, and love, one, two, three, four, and now exhaling peace, joy, and love, one, two, three, four, sending love and light into the world.

Imagine there is a beam of pure white light coming down through the top of your head. Feel that light moving through your head, into your eyes, your nose, your jaw.

Continue to breathe in peace and healing, as the light moves down, down, down, through your neck and shoulders, into your arms, your elbows, your wrists, hands, and fingertips, and continues flowing down into your collarbone, moving down your spine and into your heart.

Continue to notice your breathing. Inhaling one, two, three, four, and exhaling, one, two, three, and four.

Feel the light as it moves into your lungs and you notice with every single breath you take you are becoming more and more relaxed.

Imagine there is a beam of pure white light coming down through the top of your head. Feel that light moving through your head, into your eyes, your nose, your jaw.

Continue to breathe in peace and healing as the light moves down, down, down through your neck and shoulders, into your arms, your elbows, your wrists, hands and fingertips, and continues flowing down into your collarbone, moving down your spine and into your heart.

Continue to notice your breathing. Inhaling one, two, three, four, and exhaling, one, two, three, and four.

Feel the light as it moves into your lungs and you notice with every single breath you take you are becoming more and more relaxed.

Continue to breathe in this loving light as it moves down, down, down toward the base of your spine, flowing into your thighs, your knees, your calves, your ankles and heels, and down into the soles of your feet and into your toes.

Imagine the light is getting stronger now as it moves from the crown of your head, all the way down through your spine, into your legs, and moves down and out the soles of your feet.

Breathe in one, two, three, four, and exhale one, two, three, four. Very good.

Notice the light becoming even stronger now, so strong it begins pouring out of your heart, creating a beautiful golden ball of light that surrounds you by about three feet in all directions. Imagine yourself floating inside this peaceful golden ball of light as you breathe in one, two, three, four, and exhale, one, two, three, four.

Notice how safe, secure, and relaxed you feel inside the golden light as you breathe in one, two, three, four, and exhale one, two, three, four. Very nice.

Know that within this healing golden light, only that which is of your highest good can come through.

Very good.

Breathe in one, two, three, four, exhale one, two, three, four. Notice how relaxed you feel. More relaxed than ever before, safe and secure within the golden light.

Go ahead and imagine there is a doorway in front of you. You can see the door, feel the door, or just have an inner knowing that there is a doorway in front of you.

When I count to three, you will walk through that door. Ready? One, two, three, opening the door.

Open the door now and walk or float inside the beautiful space that you love and enjoy. Find yourself back inside your Happy Place where you've been before.

Take a deep breath in through your nose, one, two, three, four, and exhale one, two, three, four as you allow yourself to become completely relaxed inside your special Happy Place. Breathe in the energy of joy, peace, and happiness as you inhale one, two, three, four, and exhale one, two, three, four. Very good.

As you start to look around your Happy Place, enjoying yourself, notice your special guide floating down from above, joining you in your Happy Place.

Say hello and notice the deep feeling of unconditional love and high regard your guide has for you. Very good. Remember, your guide is a helper who has been with you for a very, very long time, and knows every single thing there is to know about you and your soul, and your soul's journey.

Breathe in through your nose, breathing in one, two, three, four, breathing in peace and healing and light and love, exhaling, one, two, three, four. Very good. Know that with every breath you take, you continue to become more and more relaxed.

Still surrounded by that golden ball of light, safe and secure, go ahead and take your guide by the hand, and the two of you will begin now to float, up, up, up, out of your Happy Place, floating higher and higher, up, up, up into the clouds. Very good!

Imagine you are floating so high in the sky that as you look down you notice something that looks or feels like a ray of sunshine below you. This ray of sunshine represents eternity, and you and your guide are floating over today.

Imagine you can look out in the direction of your future, whichever way that is, and notice how bright your future is. Good job!

Next, imagine you can look back toward your past. In a moment, when I count to three, you and your guide will begin to float back over your past to a very early time in your soul's history, before your current lifetime. Ready?

One, two, three, floating back through eternity, going way, way, way back beyond your birth, further and further back, to the source event, the very first time or the most significant event when your soul felt anger. You will easily travel back to the source event of your anger in a time long, long ago.

When I count to three, you will arrive at this source event. One, floating back in time, two, further and further, and three, you're there. Be there now.

Recognize that source event, and as you do, imagine your guide is showing you a screen and you can watch a video and notice what is happening that made you feel anger.

What year is this, the first thing that comes to your mind?

Where are you and what's happening? Imagine it is easy to notice.

What happened to cause you anger?

What lessons did you learn in this early time?

How is this situation affecting you in your current life?

Imagine it is easy to receive this information, and as you do, notice there is an energetic cord connecting you with this event. In a moment, when I count to three, your guide will cut that cord for you, **Eliminating** unwanted energies. Ready? One, two, three, cutting the cord.

Your guide **Lightens** the area by sending you a beautiful healing light that is coming down from above, bathing the situation in peace and love, healing you and all people connected to this event.

Take a moment while this healing energy refreshes you and notice how much better you feel.

Good job.

Integrate this healing now by easily understanding what lessons you learned from this experience. Take a moment to consider what happened and why you felt anger. Have you had similar experiences in your current lifetime? How are these experiences from your past affecting you in your current lifetime? Imagine it is easy to notice. Very good.

What can you learn from this? Do you feel you can use this experience to help you now? Take your time and think of all the ways you can benefit from your new perspective. Nice job.

Allow this information to **Energize** *you as you and your guide float all the way back from this early time in eternity all the way back to today, allowing all events between then and now to realign themselves in light of this new healing. Very good.*

Having healed anger, turn and look out toward the direction of your future in your current life. Still surrounded by golden light, holding your guide's hand, notice now how much lighter and brighter your future is because of this new information and healing. Very good.

In a moment, when I count to three, you and your guide will float out into a moment in your current-life **Future** *where you are happy, healthy, and you have successfully found RELIEF from your anger.*

Ready? One, floating out into the future, two, further and further, and three, you're there. Be there now.

What year is this?

What are you doing?

How do you feel in the future?

What's happening?

How has your life changed now that you have healed your anger? Take a moment to really feel the joyous energy of this wonderful time. As you do, take a deep breath in, one, two, three, four, breathing in love and healing; exhaling, one, two, three, four. Very good.

Bring that peaceful energy with you as you take your guide's hand and the two of you begin to float back toward today, feeling pure joy, free of the feelings of anger.

When I count down from three, you will be back, once again, floating over today. Three, two, and one, you're back. Good job!

Still surrounded by golden light, holding your guide's hand, imagine the two of you begin to float down, down, down, back through the clouds until you are once again back in your Happy Place. Be there now, in your Happy Place, feeling refreshed and better than you did before.

From here, ask your guide for any further clarity or insights you need about the healing you received today.

When you're finished, imagine you can thank your guide for being here today and watch your guide float up, up, up, back to where they came from. Know that you will see your guide again soon.

Take a deep breath in through your nose, one, two, three, four, and exhale one, two, three, four, as you allow yourself to become completely relaxed inside your special Happy Place. Breathe in the energy of joy, peace, and happiness as you inhale one, two, three, four, and exhale love and light, one, two, three, four. Very good.

Turn around now and walk back through the door, back where you started your journey.

In a moment, as I count down from five, you will come back into the room, feeling awake, refreshed, and better than you did before.

Five—grounded, centered, and balanced

Four—continuing to process this new energy in your dreams tonight so by tomorrow morning, you will be fully integrated into these new insights

Three—still surrounded by that beautiful golden ball of light, knowing only that which is of your highest good can come through, you will find yourself driving carefully and being careful in all activities

Two—grounded, centered, and balanced, and

One—you're back!

How did you do? Write any insights in your healing journal. Did you discover something new about yourself? Were there any connections between your past life and current life that you noticed? What were they? Do you believe the anger is fully resolved or do you need more healing?

If you find greater healing is needed, you can always do this process again, or you could return to the cord-cutting exercise in the last section and imagine the source of your anger is out in front of you. Cut the cords as many times as needed and fill yourself with loving light. Over time and with patience, you will feel better.

Another possibility is you will uncover deeper-rooted issues that are related to challenges in your current life, and if you do the journey again you might either receive further insight from the lifetime you visited, or you may discover you go somewhere else entirely to another relevant past life and wind up deepening your overall healing. Great job for going through the journey. Remember that these processes are like an onion—you will peel back the complex layers to get to the root over time.

Whenever you delve into the deep past, you may notice more dreams begin to come up that relate to what you just uncovered, so take note, and keep your journal near the nightstand just in case. You never know what will come up.

Let's continue on.

Clearing Past Life Sadness

There is often much sadness in our world. When dealing with sadness, often you'll find your source event relates to some form of grief. Causes of grief can include the loss of a loved one, the end of a relationship that your soul had high hopes for, or even moving away to a new place and leaving familiar surroundings behind. Some souls I've worked with will even experience a deep despair for the state of humanity as a whole—which, at times, I can't say I blame them.

Grief is a deep emotion that often takes a while to relieve. I had a major breakthrough on healing grief in my current life by finding out that the person who passed away had died during my lifetimes in many other lives. That insight brought me acceptance and through that, I healed my sadness.

You might run into someone from your current life who crossed over if you have indeed known them before in a past life, or you could get a surprise along the way. Just know that whatever is for your highest good will emerge and you will ultimately be better for taking the journey.

Whatever causes your sadness, honor it. Your guide is going to assist you in returning to the strongest event and can prove quite comforting when you're there, bringing a calming light over the situation to ease your soul. With that in mind, let's get started.

For the first part of your journey, hopefully you've made some recordings that guide you into your Happy Place where you meet your guide and float into the sky. This journey will begin once you're already there and about to go into your past. Refer back to the first exercise in this chapter on "Clearing Past Life Anger" for the complete text for the beginning of your journey. Let's begin!

Exercise
. . . .

Having found your spirit guide, the two of you float out above the current day and time. Go ahead now and imagine looking out in the direction of your future, whichever way that is, and notice how bright your future is. Good job!

Next, imagine you can look back toward your past. In a moment, when I count to three, you and your guide will begin to float back over your past to a very early time in your soul's history, before your current lifetime. Ready?

One, two, three, floating back through eternity, going way, way, way back beyond your birth, further and further back, to the source event, the very first time or the most significant event when your soul ever felt sadness. You will easily travel back to the source event of your sadness to a time long, long ago.

When I count to three, you will arrive at this source event. One, floating back in time, two, further and further, and three, you're there. Be there now.

Recognize that source event, and as you do, imagine seeing a video that shows why you feel sadness.

What year is this, the first thing that comes to your mind?

Where are you and what's happening? Imagine it is easy to notice.

What happened to cause you sadness?

What lessons did you learn in this early time?

How is this situation affecting you in your current life?

Imagine it is easy to receive this information, and as you do, notice there is an energetic cord connecting you with this event. In a moment,

*when I count to three, your guide will cut that cord for you, **Eliminat-**
ing unwanted energies. Ready? One, two, three, cutting the cord.*

*Your guide **Lightens** the area by sending healing light that bathes
the situation in peace and love, healing everyone connected to this event.
Feel this healing light moving into every single cell in your body, healing and relieving you.*

*Integrate this loving energy and allow the healing light to relieve
your sadness. If you need to cry, that is fine. Know that as you release
tears, you are feeling better and better, and soon you will be lighter than
before. Thinking about the source of your sadness, how does that relate
to your current life? How can you use this information to improve your
situation? Can you accept the past better now? Or deepen a connection
with a loved one? What specific learning did your soul choose through
this experience? Imagine you easily remember what lessons you learned
from this experience. How are these past events affecting your current
lifetime? Imagine it is easy to notice. Very good.*

*Allow this knowledge to **Energize** and empower you as you and
your guide float back to today, allowing all events between then and
now to heal. Very good.*

*Having healed sadness, holding your guide's hand, float into your
current-life **Future** where you are happy, healthy, and you have successfully found RELIEF from your sadness.*

Ready? Be there now.

What year is this?

What are you doing?

How do you feel in the future?

What's happening?

*How has your life changed now that you have healed your sadness?
Very good.*

*Feel the joyous energy of this wonderful time, breathing in love and
healing, and exhaling, one, two, three, four. Very good.*

*Bring that peaceful feeling with you as you float back toward today,
free of the feelings of sadness.*

*When I count down from three, you will be floating over today.
Three, two, and one, you're back. Good job!*

Surrounded by a protective golden light, find your Happy Place, and ask your guide for further clarity about the healing you received today. When you're finished, thank your guide and watch your guide float back to where they came from.

Take a deep breath in through your nose, one, two, three, four, and exhale one, two, three, four. Breathe in the energy of joy, peace, and happiness as you inhale one, two, three, four, and exhale love and light, one, two, three, four. Very good.

Turn around now and walk back through the door where you started your journey.

When I count down from five, you will come back into the room, feeling awake, refreshed, and better than you did before.

Five—grounded, centered, and balanced

Four—continuing to process this new energy in your dreams tonight so by tomorrow morning, you will be fully integrated into these new insights

Three—still surrounded by that beautiful golden ball of light, knowing that only that which is of your highest good can come through, you will find yourself driving carefully and being careful in all activities

Two—grounded, centered, and balanced, and

One—you're back!

How did you do on that exercise? Any deeper insights? Were you able to find some RELIEF from sadness? Grief and sadness are very complex emotions that take time to heal, so go easy on yourself and know that your healing is unfolding in divine time. This is another process you may want to go through more than once. You may find the journey to be reminiscent of something you'd already considered before, or there may be new insights or even new places where sadness lingers in your subconscious, so take your time and know all is well.

Hopefully by now the processes are becoming more routine. You are learning through repetition how to go down the road in the journey to get where you need to go, so each time you use the process, more will be revealed. Journaling about your insights can be quite helpful for letting those feelings out completely. Nice job!

What past lives have you experienced so far? Were you surprised?

Many clients are not surprised at all by their experiences because much of the time our prior incarnations are in places we've been fascinated with throughout our lives. The regression helps put those interests into greater perspective.

Hopefully, aside from the interesting self-discoveries you've made thus far, you've also felt some energetic releases with regard to some of the heavier energies possibly weighing you down. With each session you embark on, that lightening of the soul becomes more profound—at least, that's what I've found for myself, and my clients have reported the same. Nice job!

Clearing Past Life Anxiety

Our next clearing will go a bit deeper into your mind as we go back and clear anxiety from your past lives. Like the prior two exercises, you may experience some surprises along the way, but hopefully by now you know upsetting feelings caused by the events from your past can be relieved. One interesting aspect about taking these journeys is that, many times, the thing you thought you resolved in your current life winds up having deep roots in the past and can show up during this next journey. The other thing that might happen is that the first time you attempt to clear your anxiety, you may only go back as far as something that troubled you deeply in your current life. Either way, be open. Anxiety is complex, so consider this an adventure, see what happens, and know all is well! Once again, please refer back to the exercise "Clearing Past Life Anger" to see the full journey. Let's begin!

Exercise
· · · · · ·

Surrounded by a loving golden light, your spirit guide joins you as the two of you float into your Happy Place and rise up, up, up into the gorgeous blue skies. The two of you find yourselves floating over today and you look in the direction of your future, whichever way that is, and notice how bright your future is. Good job!

Next, imagine you can look back toward your past. In a moment, when I count down from three, you and your guide will begin to float back over your past to a very early time in your soul's history, before your current lifetime, to the source of your anxiety during a time long, long ago. You will go to the very first time, or the most significant time your soul ever felt anxiety, and on the count of three you will be there. One, two, and three, you're there. Be there now.

Recognize that source event; watch a video that shows what happened to create anxiety.

What year is this, the first thing that comes to your mind?

Where are you and what's happening? Imagine it is easy to notice.

What happened to cause you anxiety?

What lessons did you learn in this early time?

How is this situation affecting you in your current life?

Imagine it is easy to receive this information, and as you do, notice the energetic cord your guide will cut now for you, **Eliminating** unwanted energies. Ready? One, two, three, cutting the cord.

Your guide **Lightens** the area with healing light that is coming down from above, bathing you in peace and love, healing all people connected to this event. Notice how much better you feel. Very good.

Integrate this information into every single cell in your body. Feel the healing becoming part of you as you easily understand the lessons you learned from this experience. How are these experiences affecting you in your current lifetime? What caused your anxiety? Is this something you deal with in your current life? What strategies did you discover to help you feel better? What change can you make right now to know you are totally free from anxiety? What lessons did your soul learn from the anxiety you released today? Take your time and allow your guide to help you gain insight into all these areas and bring you support and loving light, then move on when you're ready.

Allow this information to **Energize** you as you and your guide come back to today.

Look toward your current-life future. Still surrounded by golden light, holding your guide's hand, float to a moment in your current-life **Future** where you are happy, healthy, and you have successfully found RELIEF from your anxiety. Ready? One, floating out into the future, two, further and further, and three, you're there. Be there now.

What year is this?

What are you doing?

How do you feel in the future?

What's happening?

How has your life changed now that you have healed your anxiety?

Very good.

Take a moment to experience joy and peace. Bring that peaceful energy with you as you float back toward today, feeling pure joy, free of the feelings of anxiety. Be there now, floating over today. Good job!

Still holding your guide's hand, float through the clouds until you are once again back in your Happy Place. Be there now. Ask for any insights you need about the healing you received today, then thank your guide for helping you. Say goodbye for now and know you will see your guide again soon.

Breathe in through your nose, one, two, three, four, and exhale one, two, three, four, and become completely relaxed inside your special Happy Place. Very good.

Go ahead now and walk back through the door where you started your journey.

In a moment, when I count down from five, you will come back into the room, feeling awake, refreshed, and better than you did before.

Five—grounded, centered, and balanced

Four—continuing to process this new energy in your dreams tonight so by tomorrow morning, you will be fully integrated into these new insights

Three—still surrounded by that beautiful golden ball of light, knowing only that which is of your highest good can come through, you will find yourself driving carefully and being careful in all activities

Two—grounded, centered, and balanced, and

One—you're back!

How did you do with that journey? Remember to take notes along the way. How did that feel? Go ahead and write down any important insights in your journal. Were you surprised by what came up, or did you deepen your understanding of something you'd already been working on?

What past lives did you uncover this time? Can you see any common themes you've had in any of the lives you've uncovered so far? For example, were you a soldier several times, or did you have certain kinds of challenges? Often the past lives that initially seem totally unrelated can have deeper connections when you look further, and all that information can lead to a total transformation for your consciousness, your life, and overall happiness.

Repeat as necessary and write about anything helpful or insightful that might deepen your experience later on. You're clearly on your journey of transformation now and I hope the adventure is going smoothly. Keep going!

Clearing Past Life Fear/Phobia

Fears can be quite challenging, particularly in past lives. Once you uncover the source of some of your earliest fears, huge transformation can occur.

We all have things we're afraid of that would benefit from some healing, so for this exercise, I want you to consciously come up with ideas for something you'd like to resolve, and set your intention beforehand so you know what you're aiming for in terms of what will be cleared. This doesn't have to be anything super traumatic either. You may be afraid of spiders because one crawled on you when you were ten, and now you wonder if there are any past life connections there. Or you may not like thunderstorms because lightning struck too close to your home when you were little and when you go into the past, lo and behold, you find out that wasn't the only time storms frightened you. You get the idea. It doesn't matter what it is as long as it's meaningful for you. Any time you do a regression you can always choose to set your intention for what you want to clear. For the fear journey, though, I think it's especially helpful. No matter how small and insignificant, I'm sure you have at least one thing you can consciously recall that bothers you, even just a little bit. You may want to glance back at your journal entries from earlier if you need to refresh your memory, or you can go on the journey and be open to whatever comes up. Either way, there's no right or wrong here.

You will view these things as if watching them on television or on your cell phone so you can grasp what's going on without the emotional charge. You will begin the journey by floating over today and connecting with your guide. Once you access your Happy Place, you and your guide will float away. As always, you can access your full script from the "Clearing Past Life Anger" process at the beginning of this chapter. With that, let's get to it!

Exercise
· · · · · · ·

Close your eyes and immediately notice you are easily surrounded by the loving golden light—safe, secure, and protected, you know only that which is of your highest good can come through. Walk through the door into your Happy Place and meet your guide. Float away together as you find yourself high up in the clouds. You are floating over today. Turn toward your future. Notice how bright your future is. Good job!

Turn toward your past. In a moment, when I count to three, you and your guide will begin to float back over your past to a very early time in your soul's history, before your current lifetime, to the source event, the very first time or the most significant event when your soul ever felt fear. Now, when I count to three, you will arrive at this source event. One, floating back in time, two, further and further, and three, you're there. Be there now.

Recognize that event, and imagine your guide shows you a screen. Watch a video and notice what happened to cause fear.

What year is this, the first thing that comes to your mind?

Where are you and what's happening? Imagine it is easy to notice.

What happened to cause you fear?

What lessons did you learn in this early time?

How is this situation affecting you in your current life?

*Notice the energetic cord connecting you with this event, and when I count to three, your guide will cut that cord for you, **Eliminating** unwanted energies. Ready? One, two, three, cutting the cord.*

*Your guide **Lightens** the area, sending a beautiful, healing light to you and all other people connected to this event. Take a moment while* *this healing energy refreshes you and notice how much better you feel. Good job.*

*   **Integrate** *the energy by asking your spirit guide to continue to send you the loving, healing light, allowing that light to completely expand every cell in your body until your fear melts away. Allow your guide to help you understand the lessons you learned. How are these experiences affecting your current lifetime? Knowing some fears keep you safe, if this fear is no longer needed anymore, would it be okay to let that go now? If so, hand that fear or any residual energy of fear over to your guide now. Allow your guide to take fear from you and throw it away. Very good. Imagine you can easily notice you are no longer affected by your fear. Very good.*

*   Allow this information to* **Energize** *you as you and your guide float back from this early time in eternity all the way back to today, allowing all events between then and now to realign themselves in light of this new healing. Very good.*

*   Having healed fear, turn toward the direction of your future in your current life. Still surrounded by golden light, holding your guide's hand, notice now how much lighter and brighter your future is because of this new information and healing. Very good.*

*   In a moment, when I count to three, you and your guide will float out into a moment in your current-life* **Future** *where you are happy, healthy, and you have successfully found* **RELIEF** *from your fear. Ready? One, floating out into the future, two, further and further, and three, you're there. Be there now.*

*   What year is this?*

*   What are you doing?*

*   How do you feel in the future?*

*   What's happening?*

*   How has your life changed now that you have healed your fear?*

*   Very good.*

*   Take a moment to really feel the joyous energy of this wonderful time. As you do, take a deep breath in, one, two, three, four, breathing in love and healing, exhaling, one, two, three, four. Bring that peaceful*

energy with you, take your guide's hand and float back toward today, free of the feelings of fear.

Still surrounded by golden light, float over today. While holding your guide's hand, imagine the two of you float down, back through the clouds to your Happy Place. Ask your guide for clarity about the healing you received.

When you're finished, thank your guide and watch them float up, back to where they came from. Allow yourself to completely relax. Breathe in joy, peace, and happiness, and exhale love and light. Very good.

Turn around and go back to where you started your journey. In a moment, when I count down from five, you will come back into the room, feeling awake, refreshed, and better than you did before.

Five—grounded, centered, and balanced

Four—continuing to process this new energy in your dreams tonight so by tomorrow morning, you will be fully integrated into these new insights

Three—still surrounded by that beautiful golden ball of light, knowing only that which is of your highest good can come through, you will find yourself driving carefully and being careful in all activities.

Two—grounded, centered, and balanced, and

One—you're back!

How did you do with that exercise? You may have more than one fear you want to clear, so if that's the case, go back and try it again with a different intention. For example, if you were afraid of spiders and you cleared that the first time, the next time you do the exercise, tell yourself that you are going to work on your dislike of snakes instead. Whatever you set your intention to clear will determine the outcome, or you could simply have your guide take you to whichever event is for your highest good, that would give you the greatest benefit at this current time in your life.

You may do this a couple times, put the book away, and come back to it a few years from now and something completely out-of-the-blue may emerge. Journaling about these fears can help bring them to the surface for clearing, so feel free to write about the experience.

How do you feel now compared to when you started the journey? Did you feel confident and safe now that you've established a deeper relationship with your spirit guide? Does the golden light remain with you and surround you during these journeys? Did you feel more confident that you could find answers? What lives did you visit and how do they relate to the current life? Any new changes you can integrate to move into a brighter future? Amazing work!

Hopefully your anxiety, fear, or phobia feels better than it did before. Go easy on yourself and allow your process to unfold gradually if necessary. Meanwhile, congratulations on taking this huge step in your healing! Good job!

Clearing Past Life Trauma

Next, we are going back to a traumatic event from your past life to do a healing. By *trauma*, I do not necessarily mean you will find anything too difficult. You can either set your intentions to work on a time you felt embarrassed beyond belief in your current life and see if that has ties to the past, or maybe you had a slight fender bender in your car that you felt worse about than you should have and that might have ties to something from farther back in your soul's history. Trauma could also describe the grief you felt at a friend's passing and you want to see if you've known them before, or the stress of changing schools and not knowing anybody.

Anything is fine to work on, as long as it made an impact on your life and emotions. You can either consciously select what you want to heal or simply allow your spirit guide to be in charge and allow something to bubble up in your mind as you go along. Either way, all is well.

Your guide will always take you to an event that is for your highest good. Something you might not have recalled for years could come up, and you may be surprised by how trivial it seems to you on one level, while on another, the event may still sting, and that's where the healing can be of great benefit.

When an event presents itself, know that your soul is ready on some level to address it because at all times, your Higher Self and guide keep you safe.

The memory appeared for a reason, so honor that, trust the process, and know that all is well.

There is no doubt in my mind that every soul has trauma from their past. That's part of the human condition. What will you uncover today? Know that whatever it is will be perfect for where you're at right now, and you can always do this again later for further insights. If you've had a chance to make recordings for yourself, great, but if not, please find the full process by referring back to the first exercise in this chapter on "Clearing Past Life Anger." Let's begin!

Exercise
· · · · · · ·

Holding your spirit guide's hand, surrounded by a loving, healing light that protects you and ensures only that which is of your highest good can come through, imagine you are floating over today. Glance toward your past. In a moment, when I count to three, you and your guide will float over your past to a very early time in your soul's history, before your current lifetime, to the source event—the very first time or the most significant event when your soul ever felt trauma. You will easily travel back to a time long, long ago. One, floating back in time, two, further and further, and three, you're there. Be there now.

Recognize that source event, and as you do, imagine your guide shows you a video and you can see what caused you trauma.

What year is this, the first thing that comes to your mind?

Where are you and what's happening? Imagine it is easy to notice.

What happened to cause you trauma?

How is this situation affecting you in your current life?

Imagine it is easy to receive this information, and as you do, notice there is an energetic cord connecting you with this event. In a moment, when I count to three, your guide will cut that cord for you, Eliminating unwanted energies. Ready? One, two, three, cutting the cord.

Your guide Lightens the area by sending you a beautiful healing light that is coming down from above, bathing the situation in peace and love, healing you and all people connected to this event.

Integrate this healing light. What caused your soul to experience trauma during this very early time in your soul's history? How is this trauma affecting you now in your current lifetime? What could you do to relieve this feeling now? What did you learn from your past trauma? How are you better as a person for having been through that experience? Know you can easily understand what your soul gained from this traumatic occurrence.

Become **Energized** as you and your guide float back from this early time in eternity all the way back to today, allowing all events between then and now to realign themselves in light of this new healing. Very good.

Having healed trauma, turn and look out toward the direction of your future in your current life. Still surrounded by golden light, holding your guide's hand, notice now how much lighter and brighter your future is because of this new information and healing. Very good.

In a moment, when I count to three, you and your guide will float out into a moment in your current-life **Future** where you are happy, healthy, and you have successfully found RELIEF from your trauma. Ready? One, floating out into the future, two, further and further, and three, you're there. Be there now.

What year is this?

What are you doing?

How do you feel in the future?

What's happening?

How has your life changed now that you have healed your trauma? Very good.

Feel the joyous energy of this wonderful time. Breathe in, one, two, three, four, breathing in love and healing, and exhaling, one, two, three, four. Very good.

Take these peaceful feelings with you and take your guide's hand. Float back toward today feeling pure joy, totally free of trauma.

When I count to three, you will be back, once again, floating over today. One, two, three, you're back. Good job!

Still surrounded by golden light, holding your guide's hand, float down, down, down through the clouds until you are back in your Happy Place, feeling refreshed and better than you did before.

Ask your guide for clarity and when you're finished, thank your guide for being here today and watch your guide float back to where they came from. Know that you will see your guide again soon.

Take a deep breath in through your nose, one, two, three, four, and exhale one, two, three, four as you allow yourself to become completely relaxed. Go ahead now and walk back through the door, back where you started your journey.

When I count down from five, you will come back into the room, feeling awake, refreshed, and better than you did before.

Five—grounded, centered, and balanced

Four—continuing to process this new energy in your dreams tonight so by tomorrow morning, you will be fully integrated into these new insights

Three—still surrounded by that beautiful golden ball of light, knowing only that which is of your highest good can come through, you will find yourself driving carefully and being careful in all activities

Two—grounded, centered, and balanced, and

One—you're back!

How do you feel? Were you surprised by what came up, or had you thought about the situation before? Write down any important thoughts or messages that came through. How will you integrate that new information into your life?

Was the journey easier to take now that you've had some practice? One thing I've learned is that even if you do this once or twice, you can put the book away for a while, years even, and then come back to it later to gain further information that can be timely and valuable for whatever you're working on at the moment. Know that healing is a journey and you've just taken an important step on your path! Congratulations!

Clearing Vows & Soul Contracts

In several of the case studies, you saw firsthand how detrimental soul contracts and vows can be. When we make agreements in our deep past that are no longer serving us, chaos and anxiety can easily erupt. This is your opportunity to find out if you've made any agreements that need to be voided. You might go on this journey and find out that no, you've never made a vow, but that would be unlikely. Our souls are so vast and we've had so many unique experiences over the centuries, surely you've made a pact or two along the way. If you have any inkling on what those vows might be about, you can always attempt to set an intention for your journey or see what comes up. As usual, enjoy the adventure as you get to know yourself better than before, and please note you can always refer back to the first exercise in this chapter on "Clearing Past Life Anger" for the complete text.

Exercise
. . . .

Close your eyes and notice your guide is with you now. The two of you are floating in the clouds over today. Very good. Imagine you can look back toward your past to a very early time in your soul's history, before your current lifetime, where you made a vow or a soul agreement. You will go to the most significant event that is most affecting your current lifetime. Ready?

Float back through eternity, going way, way, way back beyond your birth, further and further back, to the source event of when you first made a vow. You will easily travel back to the time when you made this vow, long, long ago.

When I count to three, you will arrive at this event. One, floating back in time, two, further and further, and three, you're there. Be there now.

Recognize *that source event, and as you do, imagine your guide is showing you a screen and you can watch a video and notice the details of your soul contract.*

What year is this, the first thing that comes to your mind?

Where are you and what's happening? Imagine it is easy to notice.

What vow did you make and to whom?

What lessons did you learn in this early time?

How is this soul contract affecting you in your current life?

*Imagine it is easy to receive this information, and as you do, notice there is an energetic cord connecting you with this event. In a moment, when I count to three, your guide will cut that cord for you, **Eliminating** unwanted energies. Ready? One, two, three, cutting the cord.*

*Your guide **Lightens** the area by sending you a beautiful healing light that is coming down from above, bathing the situation in peace and love, healing you and all people connected to this event.*

***Integrate** this healing now. Understand how this vow affects your current life. What happened as a result of your vow? How will your life change for the better now that you have recognized this? Is it in your best interest to keep your vow, or release it? Imagine it is easy to notice. Very good.*

*Allow this information to **Energize** you as you and your guide float back to today, allowing all events between then and now to realign themselves in light of this new decision you've made regarding this vow. Having been released from this soul agreement or having renegotiated the agreement for the better, turn and look out toward your future in your current life. Surrounded by golden light, float to a moment in your current-life **Future** where you are happy, healthy, and you have successfully found RELIEF from releasing your vow.*

Ready? One, floating out into the future, two, further and further, and three, you're there. Be there now.

What year is this?

What are you doing?

How do you feel in the future?

How has your life changed now that you released or altered your soul agreement?

Bring that peaceful energy with you as you take your guide's hand and the two of you begin to float back toward today feeling pure joy, free of the unwanted influences of this vow.

When I count down from three, you will be back, once again, floating over today. Three, two, one, you're back. Good job!

Holding your guide's hand, imagine the two of you begin to float down, down, down, back through the clouds until you are back in your Happy Place. Be there now, feeling refreshed and better than you did before. Ask your guide any questions about the new decision you made today.

When you're finished, thank your guide. Watch your guide float away. Breathe in through your nose, one, two, three, four, and exhale one, two, three, four. Become completely relaxed inside your special Happy Place. Turn around now and walk back through the door, back to where you started your journey.

In a moment, when I count down from five, you will come back into the room, feeling awake, refreshed, and better than you did before.

Five—grounded, centered, and balanced

Four—continuing to process this new energy in your dreams tonight so by tomorrow morning, you will be fully integrated into these new insights

Three—still surrounded by that beautiful golden ball of light, knowing that only that which is of your highest good can come through, you will find yourself driving carefully and being careful in all activities

Two—grounded, centered, and balanced, and

One—you're back!

How did your vow-clearing session go? Did you make a vow or promise in the past? If so, did you discover that was a good thing to do, or did you decide to clear it out for your highest good? Were you surprised? Make notes on any important issue that came up, and as always, if needed, do the journey again.

Another variation of the vows journey would be going into the past to clear a curse. Over the course of what's turned out to be quite an eclectic career, I've helped hundreds of people who believed they were cursed. Curses, like vows, are often carried over from many lifetimes and can be cleared in the same way as vows by using that same journey and setting your intention to go into the past and see if you are influenced by any curses.

Of course, like much of this book, if you think you're blessed, you are, and if you don't, well…you can create a self-fulfilling prophecy, so while I feel compelled to mention that here, know you can use any of these journeys by setting your intention if you need to clear something that deep from your past. If you feel this is you and you've had the evil eye placed on you in a prior lifetime, carry that thought in mind and go through this experience again to see what comes up. Remember, soul healing comes in layers. With soul contracts, vows, and even with curses, at some point the soul signed up to experience them, so although there could be quite a lot of work to do in this area, once you do a little clearing and gratefully acknowledge the lessons and, believe it or not, the actual benefits you received from your hex, you become free to enjoy life to the fullest. Everything you experience, even unpleasant events, can ultimately be seen as a beneficial gift to facilitate soul growth. Likewise, by clearing your vows and promises, you now have a clean slate before you to go make new agreements. Or not. It's all up to you to decide.

Future Memories & Symbols

A big part of the RELIEF Method exercises involved clearing out old energies to make way for a brighter, more empowered future thanks to what you've left behind. You glimpsed your future to see how your current life changed for the better after releasing old energies of anger, fear, anxiety, and the like.

Now I'd like you to pull out your journal again and take a look back on all the thoughts and ideas you've come up with since embarking on this journey. What are you doing in life now, versus what you want to be doing in the future? What affirmations are you using? What mantras are you repeating about what you want to create this time around?

In this next exercise, you will venture back into the realm of your Future Memories so you can stay there a little longer and further experience the highest ideal for your life. You will be able to gain great insights into where you live, what you're doing as your vocation, whom you're with, and most importantly—*how you feel*. Happiness and joy are the ultimate goals. You will visit a Future Memory where you have successfully found your bliss and calling in life.

I will also ask you to come up with symbols, or visual cues, to remind you of your ultimate Happy Place so you can easily navigate your way there in the coming days, weeks, months, and years. Once you discover your special symbol that represents the life you truly want, you'll have another tool to guide you daily along your path.

Symbols are common in energy healing. They serve as shortcuts for your subconscious mind. These days, symbols are easy to explain. Just take a look at your cell phone and you're bound to see plenty of symbols—the emojis—that represent all kinds of emotions ranging from happiness, sadness, excitement. Having an image that symbolically represents your ideal life will help you move in the direction you truly want to go.

This exercise is a bit different from the earlier exercises to access your current-life future. Try them both and see which you prefer. Let's get started.

Exercise
· · · · · · ·

Begin by breathing in peace and healing, exhaling tension. Allow your breath to be balanced and nurturing throughout this journey and know with each breath you take, you feel more and more relaxed.

Go ahead now and surround yourself in a healing golden light. Knowing you are safe, you see the doorway to your Happy Place in front of you. Open that door now. Meet with your loving guide and hold their hand as the two of you begin now to float up, up, up into the air, and find yourself floating now above the light, above today.

Think about your soul's journey for a moment. All you've learned so far about yourself, where you've been, what you've done. Imagine feeling an immense sense of gratitude for all that brought you to this particular moment in time. Very good.

If you wish, you may ask your guide to provide any further insights into your soul's purpose and mission on Earth for your current life. Take your time. Ask questions and receive clarity. Very good.

Now, when I count to three, you and your guide will float out to a moment in your current-life Future where you are involved in your ideal vocation, living where you want, and experiencing life with the right people who support you in every way. In this future event, you are happier and more at ease within yourself than you have ever been before, and you know you have successfully made the necessary changes to live the life of your dreams.

Ready? One, floating out into the future, two, further and further, and three, you're there. Be there now.

What year is this?

Where are you?

Who are you with?

How do you feel?

What work are you doing and how do you know this is what you were meant to do? Imagine noticing what people tell you about your contributions and gifts. Very good.

Take a moment to really feel the joyous energy of this wonderful time. As you do, imagine you can remember back to all the steps you took to bring you to this current state of peace and joy. Notice the first step you took to create this ideal life for yourself. Very good. And then what did you do next? Imagine you can easily recall these steps because they've already happened.

Go ahead and allow every single cell in your body to expand and relax into this new energy of happiness, beginning with the tips of your toes, moving into your feet, your legs, up your spine. Cells are expanding and relaxing, allowing greater light and love to flow in and totally aligning themselves with this greater sense of peace and purpose. That light moves into your heart, joyfully opening your heart to love, as it moves into your neck, shoulders, arms, hands, and fingers and up into your mind.

As the light continues to move into all your cells, imagine your subconscious mind can give you a symbol that represents this new feeling of joy and happiness you have now.

Allow that symbol to pop into your mind's eye, or your guide may tell you what that is, or you may have an inner knowing of your symbol. Notice your symbol now and know that anytime during your life's journey when you see this symbol in the outer world, on a video, in your cell phone, or if it simply pops into your mind, you will know and recognize this as a sign that you are moving in the right direction, and all is well. Bring that new sense of love and purpose along with you as you take your guide's hand and the two of you begin to float back toward today. When I count down from three, you will be back, once again, floating over today. Three, two, and one, you're back. Good job!

Still surrounded by golden light, holding your guide's hand, imagine the two of you begin to float down, down, down, back through the clouds until you are once again back in your Happy Place. Be there now, in your Happy Place, feeling refreshed and better than you did before.

Thank your guide as they float up and away. Notice the incredible feeling of love you have in every cell in your body. Good job.

Turn around now and walk back through the door, back where you started your journey.

In a moment, when I count down from five, you will come back into the room, feeling awake, refreshed, and better than you did before.

Five—grounded, centered and balanced

Four—continuing to process this new energy in your dreams tonight so by tomorrow morning, you will be fully integrated into this new feeling of purpose and love

Three—still surrounded by that beautiful golden ball of light, knowing that anytime you see or experience the symbol you received today, you will be instantly brought back to the higher sense of peace and purpose of your brightest future and will easily move in that direction

Two—grounded, centered, and balanced, and

One—you're back!

How did that go? Did you receive new information different from what you'd experienced in the earlier exercises? Tapping into Future Memories can be one of the most powerful processes you will ever do in terms of recreating your experience. I highly recommend writing down what you received and perhaps going on your cell phone to find an applicable emoji or utilize other visual means to see if you can find an image that looks like the symbol your subconscious mind came up with today. I'd put that symbol on my mirror, in my documents, use it as a screensaver—put it anywhere you can as a reminder and encouragement. By having the image in front of you as much as possible, your unconscious mind receives a powerful signal to keep going though challenges and reminds you of your amazing personal power.

Next, put all the tools together—the breathing, clearing out unwanted energies, working with a trusted guide who loves you, visiting a Happy Place where you feel safe and supported, working with daily affirmations and positive messages, and reminding yourself that you can do whatever you put your mind to by visualizing your symbol and moving forward. With your new, expanded perspective, the sky's the limit to what you can accomplish. I'm proud of you for making it through the book and I wish you great success on your life path.

CONCLUSION

Paving the Way for Your Brightest Future

THROUGHOUT THE BOOK YOU'VE been on a journey to dig deep into your soul and into your past to shift and change things for the better. The bigger picture for why anyone would do regression work in the first place all comes down to your life in the present moment, your acceptance of yourself, and your newfound courage to empower yourself with what you've learned so you can pave the way toward a happier, brighter, and more productive future.

Happiness is the goal, and while life is not perfect, through small inner changes and continual shifts, your soul can navigate the waters of life and move in the direction that will take you to where you truly want to go.

With the painfully intense levels of anxiety, depression, and trauma so prevalent in society today, there is no better time for you to be reading this book and working on healing yourself. We are at a critical junction in our human existence, and I know with some focused attention and effort, we can overcome all the obstacles we now face.

One reason I've considered for why so many are suffering anxiety and depression now is that we are collectively and empathetically picking up on the energies of the larger world around us. We all feel for others, whether we're consciously aware of that or not. Haven't you ever talked to someone who told you something sad that happened to them and you felt bad for them? We've all had that happen because we're all connected.

That's one of the many reasons why doing hypnotic journey work is such a great tool for calming stress. When you center yourself and create healing ideas and thoughts, regardless of the swirl of chaos surrounding you in the outer world, the space around you physically shifts and transforms as you change, and life becomes more peaceful. That state of serenity then begins to ripple out to others. It's a wonderful thing to do.

Buddhists believe that it is good to dedicate one's spiritual practice to the benefit of all sentient beings by remembering that all of us, regardless of our backgrounds, have one common goal—to be happy and to avoid suffering. I think that's true. So when you heal and let go of past suffering, resentment, anger, or any other unproductive state, you are actually helping us all, and that effect ripples through the universe, through all eternity, and transforms all time—past, present, and future.

While researching this book, I found the most common emotion my clients experienced was fear. Anxiety and trauma in particular are directly linked to the experience of feeling insecure about the continuation of life. While I have collected thousands of case histories over the course of my twenty year career, many of those featured in Meet Your Karma interestingly involved people struggling with basic survival.

You may have heard of something called Maslow's Hierarchy of Needs.[10] The concept is simple—there are five levels of existence that all humans experience. The lowest level involves the quest for food and shelter. Obviously, you can't become enlightened if you're starving to death. Capital punishment for stealing food featured in many of my cases, was sadly quite common in ancient times. Wars, battles and other violent deaths also proved prevalent in cases of anxiety and trauma. It should come as no surprise that people experiencing deeper levels of past life anxiety feared death and their pain carried over into their current lifetimes.

· · · · · · · · · · · · ·

10. Saul McLeod, "Maslow's Hierarchy of Needs." Updated 2018, Simply Psychology.org, https://www.simplypsychology.org/maslow.html.

Another perhaps more surprising emotion prevalent among my clients that many people feel regarding their anxiety and panic attacks is shame. People who see themselves as part of the spiritual community often feel that they should somehow know better than to react in what they falsely believe are such unenlightened ways. Believe me, I get it. I've certainly beaten myself up plenty of times over the years. It pains me deeply to see my clients being so hard on themselves though, because you know what? We have nothing to be ashamed of! No one should apologize for having strong and often overwhelming reactions to the stressors and traumas that happen in daily life. Our feelings demonstrate our innate humanity and prove we care about our world and each other.

Remember, it takes great courage to look at yourself and work through trauma and anxiety, and yet the rewards are tremendous in terms of your future happiness and contentment.

The old saying that *it's not what happens to you but what you do about what happens* is true. Aren't you doing your best? I know I am, and I truly believe that most people in this world are simply doing their best at any given moment with the information they've been given at the time.

My clients never cease to amaze me with their stories of courage, grace, forgiveness, and wisdom when faced with unbelievable challenges. I am in constant awe of their courage and have the deepest respect for anyone who can keep going in the face of harsh adversity.

The happiest people are those who can move forward, let go of the past, and take their personal power into their own hands for the betterment of their souls. Once that shift in consciousness happens, soul growth and learning occur. You get the lesson and your soul won't go through those things again. That's what happened for me, and for so many others.

Using hypnosis and the power of the subconscious mind to recreate your personal history is the very best way I've found to shape your life into something positive and move forward with grace, no matter where you've been or what you've been through. The journey isn't always easy, but the effort is so worth the time.

The saying that *we are all one* is true. Did you know when you heal, forgive, let go, and transform yourself, you are actually doing that for all mankind from the past, present, and future? It's true! When you take the time and put in the effort to help yourself, you enrich that collective unconscious Carl Jung wrote about by creating a new way of being that others can ultimately tap into and benefit from. Any time we choose love over hate, healing and forgiveness over resentment, then we open up a new space to allow every other being who ever existed now, in the past or in the future, to do the same. We consciously co-create and shift that collective unconscious to a lighter, more loving energy that will be better for all concerned, and you are a big part of that change.

Know that I am cheering you on from the sidelines. Keep going! Keep working to understand yourself and you will find the light at the end of the tunnel that you've been seeking. You deserve to have a happy life no matter what! With that, I send you light and many blessings on your journey. Namaste!

Bibliography

Ambardekar, Nayana, M.D. "Progressive Muscle Relaxation for Stress and Insomnia." WebMD, January 20, 2018. https://www.webmd.com/sleep-disorders/muscle-relaxation-for-stress-insomnia.

Amen, Daniel G., M.D. *Change Your Brain Change Your Life: The Breakthrough Program for Conquering Anxiety, Depression, Obsessiveness, Anger and Impulsiveness.* New York: Three Rivers Press, 1998.

American Psychiatric Association. *Diagnostic and Statistical Manual of Mental Disorders. 5th ed.* Arlington, Virginia: American Psychiatric Association, 2013.

Arts & Entertainment Television. *Hoarders,* https://www.aetv.com/shows/hoarders.

Associated Press. "Poll: Nearly 8 in 10 Americans Believe in Angels." CBS News.com, December 23, 2011. https://www.cbsnews.com/news/poll-nearly-8-in-10-americans-believe-in-angels/.

Baines, John R. and Peter F. Dorman. "Ancient Egyptian Religion." Encyclopaedia Britannica, Inc., October 10, 2017. https://www.britannica.com/topic/ancient-Egyptian-religion/The-cult.

Bernstein, Morey. *The Search for Bridey Murphy.* New York, NY: Doubleday, 1989.

Bourne, Edmund PhD, and Lorna Garano. *Coping with Anxiety: 10 Ways to Relieve Anxiety, Fear & Worry, Revised Second Edition*. Oakland, CA: New Harbinger Publications, Inc., 2016.

Brogan, Kelly, M.D. and Kristin Loberg. *A Mind of Your Own: The Truth About Depression and How Women Can Heal Their Bodies to Reclaim Their Lives*. New York, NY: Harper Wave, 2016.

Collins, Robert M., William Moore and Rick Doty. "The Zeta Reticuli Star System." UFO Conspiracy.com, 1991. http://www.ufoconspiracy.com/reports/zetareticuli_star_sys.htm.

De Silva, Padma and Stanley Rachman. *Obsessive-Compulsive Disorder: The Facts, Third Edition*. New York, NY: Oxford University Press, 2004.

Dowling, Austin. "Conclave," Catholic Answers, https://www.catholic.com/encyclopedia/conclave.

Downs, Alan, PhD. *The Half-Empty Heart: A Supportive Guide to Breaking Free from Chronic Discontent*. New York, NY: St. Martin's Griffin, 2003.

Eisler, Melissa. "Learn the Ujjayi Breath, An Ancient Yogic Breathing Technique." Chopra.com, https://chopra.com/articles/learn-the-ujjayi-breath-an-ancient-yogic-breathing-technique.

Foa, Edna B., PhD, and Linda Wasmer Andrews. *If Your Adolescent has an Anxiety Disorder: An Essential Resource for Parents*. New York, NY: Oxford University Press, 2006.

Forward, Susan, PhD, and Craig Buck. *Obsessive Love: When It Hurts Too Much to Let Go*. New York, NY: Bantum Books, 1991.

Frost, Randy O. *Compulsive Hoarding and the Meaning of Things*. Boston, MA: Mariner Books, Houghton Mifflin Harcourt, 2011.

Gardner, James, M.D. and Arthur H. Bell, PhD. *Phobias and How to Overcome Them: Understanding and Beating Your Fears*. Newburyport, MA: New Page Books, 2005.

Gecewicz, Claire. "'New Age' Beliefs Common Among Religious, Non-religious Americans." Pew Research Center, October 1, 2018. http://www.pewresearch.org/fact-tank/2018/10/01/new-age-beliefs-common-among-both-religious-and-nonreligious-americans/.

Greenspan, Jesse. "8 Things You May Not Know About the Papal Conclave: As Cardinals Gather in Rome to Elect a New Pontiff, Take a Glimpse Inside the Famously Secretive Papal Conclave." History.com, March11, 2013. https://www.history.com/news/8-things-you-may-not-know-about-the-papal-conclave.

Harvey, Ian. "Europeans in the Middle Ages Believed Lice Were a Sign of Good Health." The VintageNews.Com, March 23, 2017. https://www.thevintagenews.com/2017/03/23/europeans-in-the-middleages-believed-that-lice-were-a-sign-of-good-health/.

Hollander, Eric, M.D. and Nicholas Bakalar. *Coping with Social Anxiety: The Definitive Guide to Effective Treatment Options.* New York: NY: Owl Books, Henry Holt & Company, 2005.

Hunt, Douglas, M.D. *What Your Doctor May Not Tell You About Anxiety, Phobias, & Panic Attacks: The All-Natural Program That Can Help You Conquer Your Fears.* New York, NY: Warner Books, 2005.

Johnston, Joni E., Psy.D. and O. Joseph Bienvenu, M.D., PhD. *Idiot's Guide to Overcoming Depression, Second Edition.* New York, NY: Alpha Books, 2014.

Jung, C.G. and R.F.C. Hull. *The Archetypes and the Collective Unconscious (Collected Works of C.G. Jung Vol. 9, Part 1).* New York, NY: Princeton University Press, Second Edition, 1981.

Maltz, Maxwell. *Psycho-Cybernetics: A New Way to Get More Living Out of Life.* New York, NY: Simon & Schuster, 1960.

Maté, Gabor, M.D. *Scattered: How Attention Deficit Disorder Originates and What You Can Do About It.* New York, NY: Dutton Books, 1999.

McLeod, Saul. "Short Term Memory." Simply Psychology.org, 2009. https://www.simplypsychology.org/short-term-memory.html.

McVey-Noble, Merry E., PhD, Sony Khemlani-Patel, PhD, and Fugen Neziroglu, PhD, ABBP, ABPP. *When Your Child is Cutting: A Parent's Guide to Helping Children Overcome Self-Injury.* Oakland, CA: New Harbinger Publications, 2006.

Miller, George A. "The Magical Number Seven, Plus or Minus Two: Some Limits on Our Capacity for Processing Information." *Psychological Review*, 63, 81-97. Harvard University, 1956. http://psychclassics. yorku.ca/Miller/.

Mollica, Richard F., M.D. *Healing Invisible Wounds: Paths to Hope and Recovery in a Violent World*. New York, NY: Hartcourt, Inc., 2006.

Moore, Clement Clarke. "A Visit from Saint Nicholas." *The Random House Book of Poetry for Children*. New York, NY: Random House, 1983.

"Mouth Breathing: Symptoms, Complications & Treatments," Healthline. com. https://www.healthline.com/health/mouth-breathing#causes.

"Nose Breathing or Mouth Breathing? What's the Correct Way to Breathe?" Breathing.com. https://breathing.com/pages/nose-breathing.

Pai, Anushka, Alina M. Suris and Carol S. North. "Posttraumatic Stress Disorder in the DSM-5: Controversy, Change, and Conceptual Consideration." MDPI, Basel, Switzerland. https://www.ncbi.nlm.nih.gov/pmc/articles/PMC5371751/.

Paxton, Matt and Phaedra Hise. *The Secret Lives of Hoarders: True Stories of Tackling Extreme Clutter*. New York, NY: Perigee Books, 2011.

Ryan, Thomas. "25 percent of US Christians believe in reincarnation. What's wrong with this picture?" AmericanMagazine.org, October 21, 2015. https://www.americamagazine.org/faith/2015/10/21/25-percent-us-christians-believe-reincarnation-whats-wrong-picture.

Sarkis, Stephanie Moulton, PhD. *10 Simple Solutions to Adult ADD: How to Overcome Chronic Distraction & Accomplish Your Goals, Second Edition*. Oakland, CA: New Harbinger Publications, Inc., 2011.

Serpa, Vincent, Fr. O.P. "Who said, 'Love the sinner, hate the sin'?" Catholic.com, August 4, 2011. https://www.catholic.com/qa/who-said-love-the-sinner-hate-the-sin.

Shakespeare, William. *Hamlet*. New York, NY: MacMillan Collector's Library, New Edition, August 23, 2016.

Stahl, Bob, PhD, and Wendy Millstine. *Calming the Rush of Panic: A Mindfulness-Based Stress Reduction Guide to Freeing Yourself from Panic Attacks & Living a Vital Life.* Oakland, CA: New Harbinger Publications, Inc., 2013.

Mental Health Resources

THANKFULLY, THROUGH THE INTERNET, finding help for various challenges in life has never been easier, as long as you have the courage to reach out and ask for what you need. Here are some links to resources I hope you'll find helpful.

American Psychiatric Association. http://www.psych.org/

American Psychological Association. https://www.apa.org/

Anxiety and Depression Association of America. http://www.adaa.org /living-with-anxiety/ask-and-learn/resources/

Anxiety Disorder Resource Center. http://www.adaa.org/living-with -anxiety/ask-and-learn/resources/

Depression and Bipolar Support Alliance. http://www.dbsalliance.org/

Mental Health Resources for Hoarders, including help for pets. https:// www.aetv.com/shows/hoarders/exclusives/treatment-resources/

National Alliance on Mental Illness. https://www.nami.org/

National Center for Complementary and Integrative Health. https:// nccih.nih.gov/

National Institutes for Heath. http://www.nlm.nih.gov/medlineplus /mentalhealth.html/

National Suicide Prevention Lifeline. 1-800-273-8255. http://www.sui cidepreventionlifeline.org/

U.S. Government Mental Health page. https://www.usa.gov/mental-health -substance-abuse/

To Write to the Author

If you wish to contact the author or would like more information about this book, please write to the author in care of Llewellyn Worldwide Ltd. and we will forward your request. Both the author and the publisher appreciate hearing from you and learning of your enjoyment of this book and how it has helped you. Llewellyn Worldwide Ltd. cannot guarantee that every letter written to the author can be answered, but all will be forwarded. Please write to:

Shelley A. Kaehr, PhD
⁒ Llewellyn Worldwide
2143 Wooddale Drive
Woodbury, MN 55125-2989

Please enclose a self-addressed stamped envelope for reply,
or $1.00 to cover costs. If outside the U.S.A., enclose
an international postal reply coupon.

Many of Llewellyn's authors have websites with additional
information and resources. For more information,
please visit our website at http://www.llewellyn.com

GET MORE AT LLEWELLYN.COM

Visit us online to browse hundreds of our books and decks, plus sign up to receive our e-newsletters and exclusive online offers.

- Free tarot readings • Spell-a-Day • Moon phases
- Recipes, spells, and tips • Blogs • Encyclopedia
- Author interviews, articles, and upcoming events

GET SOCIAL WITH LLEWELLYN

Find us on 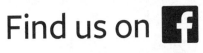 🐦 @LlewellynBooks

www.Facebook.com/LlewellynBooks

GET BOOKS AT LLEWELLYN

LLEWELLYN ORDERING INFORMATION

 Order online: Visit our website at www.llewellyn.com to select your books and place an order on our secure server.

Order by phone:
- Call toll free within the US at 1-877-NEW-WRLD (1-877-639-9753)
- We accept VISA, MasterCard, American Express, and Discover.

 Order by mail:
Send the full price of your order (MN residents add 6.875% sales tax) in US funds plus postage and handling to: Llewellyn Worldwide, 2143 Wooddale Drive, Woodbury, MN 55125-2989

POSTAGE AND HANDLING

STANDARD (US): (Please allow 12 business days)
$30.00 and under, add $6.00.
$30.01 and over, FREE SHIPPING.

CANADA:
We cannot ship to Canada. Please shop your local bookstore or Amazon Canada.

INTERNATIONAL:
Customers pay the actual shipping cost to the final destination, which includes tracking information.

Visit us online for more shipping options.
Prices subject to change.

FREE CATALOG!

To order, call
1-877-
NEW-WRLD
ext. 8236
or visit our
website

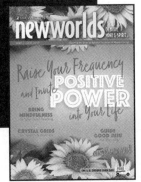